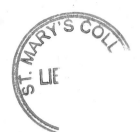

Hearing Differently
The Impact of
Hearing Impairment on Family Life

Heard melodies are sweet, but those unheard
Are sweeter; therefore, ye soft pipes, play on;
Not to the sensual ear, but, more endear'd
Pipe to the spirit ditties of no tone.

John Keats, 'Ode to a Grecian Urn'

Hearing Differently
The Impact of Hearing Impairment on Family Life

RUTH A. MORGAN-JONES, PHD.

W
WHURR PUBLISHERS
LONDON AND PHILADELPHIA

© 2001 Whurr Publishers Ltd
First published 2001
by Whurr Publishers Ltd
19b Compton Terrace
London N1 2UN England and
325 Chestnut Street, Philadelphia PA 19106 USA

British Library Cataloguing in Publication Data

A catalogue record for this book
is available from the British Library.

ISBN 1 86156 177 6

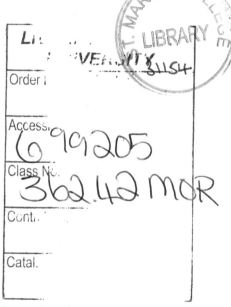
Printed and bound in the UK by Athenaeum Press Ltd,
Gateshead, Tyne & Wear.

Contents

Foreword

The great American sociologist Robert Ezra Park recalled in old age the impact which William James had made upon him as a student at Harvard at the end of the nineteenth century:

> William James read us one day his essay on 'A certain blindness in human beings.' I was greatly impressed at the time, and, as I have reflected upon it since, the ideas suggested there have assumed a steadily increasing significance.
>
> The 'blindness' of which James spoke is the blindness which each of us is likely to have for the meaning of other people's lives. At any rate what sociologists most need to know is what goes on behind the faces of men, what it is that makes life for each of us either dull or thrilling. For 'if you lose the joy, you lose all'. The thing that gives zest to life or makes life dull is, however, as James says, 'a personal secret' which has, in every single case, to be discovered. Otherwise we do not know the world in which we actually live
>
> (Park, 1950: vi–vii)

Social scientists seek to throw light on the human condition by making people's personal worlds intelligible to someone who does not live in that world. They can make known to the general reader the conditions of existence of those whose lives are often hidden or unknown.

Dr R.A. Morgan-Jones's study of the impact of hearing impairment on family life is a fine example of such an approach. *Hearing Differently*, moreover, goes beyond conventional studies of the impact of disability. How do families where one partner is deafened and the other is not manage their world? How is disability experienced both by the disabled person, and by their hearing partner? Drawing upon the influential anthropological ideas of Elizabeth Bott, Dr Morgan-Jones explores the dynamics and networks which bind couples together in families, and how these work out in the marital relationship where one partner has a hearing impairment.

This book is based upon sensitive case studies. One place to start reading the book is at the end in Appendix B, with the short profiles of the 11 couples and five individuals whose experiences form the basis of this study. The people purposely represent a comprehensive range with reference to the degree and time of onset of their hearing loss. Some were born with their loss while the majority acquired theirs in either childhood or later life. Most, but not all, were able to obtain a good education. The experience of hearing differently and learning to negotiate one's unique journey stands out from her matter of fact descriptions. Dr Morgan-Jones is a fine researcher whose serial interviews lay before us the experiences of couples talking with remarkable frankness about what it is like to cope with hearing differently, and to bring up children who must adapt to one parent being deaf. There is much to learn here also about how families cope creatively with adversity. At the same time, the book takes us away from simplistic division of the world into 'the hearing' and 'the deaf' and provides a much more positive picture of how people cope and adapt than is usual in discussions of social problems and social disadvantage.

Nor does the author shrink from addressing the social policy issues which a major disability such as hearing impairment raises. Numerically a large minority of the population are affected, particularly older people. Between 15 and 20 per cent of the population suffer from hearing impairment, yet many misapprehensions exist about the social circumstances of people affected by hearing loss. These policy concerns are not, however, abstractions, but are continually brought back to the personal and family circumstances of those who were interviewed for the study. Their voices speak to us through Dr Morgan-Jones's vital analysis of human experience.

Martin Bulmer
Foundation Fund Professor of Sociology
University of Surrey, UK

Acknowledgements

This book would not have been written without the whole-hearted courageous cooperation of the 11 couples and five single people who shared their lives so generously with me. Ten interview sessions over a six-month period is a big commitment to give a social researcher. I felt very privileged to be part of the lives of these families during this time. In order to protect their identities, I have given them all different names and made slight alterations to other details of their lives and histories. It is my hope that they will find this book of interest and in hindsight be glad of their trust in me.

I am indebted to Nina Cohen, marital therapist at the Tavistock Institute of Marital Studies. With great skill and sensitivity she guided my transition from counsellor to researcher. Simultaneously I began working with Sally Sainsbury at the London School of Economics in the Department of Social Policy. Ten years is a long time to work with one person and I always found Sally patient, clear headed and wise. I am particularly grateful for her encouragement to use methodology devised by Elizabeth Bott, *Families and Social Network*, as it made possible the discovery of new ground in my own work.

I was also inspired by the pioneers in my field, both hearing and deaf, not only in the UK but also in the USA, Germany and Turkey. During the course of my developing work, I was able to meet and talk with Rocky Stone, Lesley Jones, Peter Wood, Carol Padden, Michael Harvey, Hilde Schlesinger, Alan Thomas, Jack Ashley, Holly Elliott, Bruce Heller, Laurel Glass and Paul Preston, all of whom encouraged me in different ways. I am particularly grateful to Helen Sloss Luey whose generous hospitality, experience and support was a much appreciated gift. I also feel a debt to Jim Kyle, Klaus Verch and Werner Richtberg who published the papers I presented at conferences, thus giving me further encouragement during the early days of my work. This encouragement was increased by Professors David Downes and Martin Bulmer, my

Ph.D. examiners, who gave me hope that my dissertation was worthy of publication.

I would also like to thank Jane and Charlie Macnaghten, Bob Beck, Dr Kari and Phil Carstairs, Rev'd Christopher and Sally Kevill-Davis, Rt Rev'd Hewlett and Joy Thompson, Rt Rev'd Michael and Lou Scott-Joynt, Rev'd Robert Ferguson, Gill and John Hinson, Janet and Stephen Davies, Elizabeth Marchant, Pat Hattersley-Smith, the Women's Workshop on Qualitative Family and Household Research, Sue Hardaker, Dr Brian and Mary Shaw, the Seamus and Yvonne Symth family, the Graham and Liz Carpenter family, the John and Dr Rosemary Fowler family, Rev'd David and Dr Sarah Frith, Rev'd Jacques and Susan Desrosier, Margaret Wilkinson, Professor Margaret and Paul Harris, Andrew Rowe, MP, Dr Sheila Rowe, Dr Pauline Waters, Jane and Michael Wearne, Barbara Reid, Ann and Ray Wallace, Trish and Neil Turrell, Dr Barbara Sirota, Dr Alan Weinstein, Sally Totenbier, Dr Gary Briggs and Dr Kent Groff for their valued support, stimulation and friendship which helped indirectly in writing the thesis and book; and in some cases, hands-on proofreading was also given.

There was also a group of North American relatives and friends who gave me unstinting hospitality throughout the ten years. These were my mother and father, Nancy and Hans Panofsky, my sister, Anne Panofsky, my aunts and uncles, 'Pief' and Adele Panofsky and Pat and Dave Riker. The support, encouragement and hospitality of enduring family friends, Andy and Susan Lipchak and Nick and Louise Hanlon has also been deeply appreciated and will always be remembered.

I am indebted to the Rt Rev'd Tom Butler, now Bishop of Southwark, who took a genuine interest in my work and shared his wisdom generously over many years. I have also been fortunate to benefit from the interest and support of Eileen Carey, wife of the Archbishop of Canterbury.

However, the person who kept the home fires burning for me at all times was my husband, Christopher, who somehow was able to hold down a very demanding job and have hot nourishing meals prepared for me on a regular basis. He has also been my most severe, but constructive critic. Likewise, my son, Edward, and daughter, Liz, have managed to be understanding with my absentmindedness when pursuing such long-term projects.

PART I

Ways of Looking at Hearing Loss and Relationships

CHAPTER 1

Introduction: the nature of the study

Introduction

Hearing Differently is about discovering the challenges in relationships when one partner has a hearing impairment, in most cases acquired, and the other hears normally. Since marriage and cohabitation cannot be seen merely in terms of a relationship between the two people involved, it must be set in the context of wider neighbour-hood relationships. The impact of hearing impairment on the inter-relationships between the couple and the wider networks is a crucial aspect of this psychosocial study.

Past marginalization of Deaf culture has naturally lead to a reaction as a consequence of which many issues such as sign language have been politicized (Harris, 1995). This qualitative/anthropological study examines another approach to the complex interaction between the hearing world, the world of those with some hearing loss and the Deaf world. The study draws attention to the fact that politicizing a problem is not the only way to manage it and makes us ask ourselves what the micro level has to teach the macro level.

Hearing Differently is also about seeing the distinction between hearing as one of the five senses necessary for the development of one's speech, education, career, and the enjoyment of many pleasures in life and the listening required in order to comprehend, to understand, and empathize. This sort of listening is not related to the physiology of one's inner ears, but is nurtured by life's experiences and a continuing dialogue between one's head and heart. It is also about knowing that intimate relationships have to be given something extra in the way of time and attention if they are to work and

3

function better and more creatively in the complex world in which we live. As one in three marriages continues to dissolve, and communication breakdown is seen to be a central factor in this process, psychological deafness in marriage (Olson, Fournier and Druckman, 1986) has become a much bigger issue than its physical cousin. However, it is doubtful that this will be for long. The RNID (Royal National Institute for the Deaf) suggests that today 7.5 million people in the UK are hearing impaired. This number is expected to rise dramatically as the growth of the numbers of elderly people in the population increases and the number of people suffering from NIHL (noise-induced hearing loss) escalates. With regard to the latter, the number of people exposed to potentially dangerous sound levels has tripled since the early eighties (*Evening Standard*, 1999). It is not at all surprising that the National Acoustics laboratory of Australia has predicted that 78 per cent of men and 25 per cent of women will be hearing impaired by the year 2015 as a partial result of NIHL. This is because men are more likely to over stimulate their ears with extraneous noise, for example, from motor cycles, boat engines and guns. Because of the macho culture which devalues safety measures, men are more likely not to wear their ear defenders when engaging in noisy occupations or when in contact with loud music. Following on from this point is the belief that the current generation of teenagers has been exposed repeatedly to higher noise levels than in the past. It is thus predicted that in a few years, there will be an epidemic of hearing loss in people in their twenties and thirties. The evidence suggests that the harmful effects of noise are cumulative and such damage to the fine hairs in the inner ear or cochlea is irreparable. By the time someone realizes they are not hearing normally, there is little the medical profession can do (*Lancet*, 1994).

Most of the people who took part in this study were specifically chosen because they are both ordinary and extraordinary in the way they managed their hearing loss. This is because many, but not all, were fortunate enough to have the resilience required (Walsh, 1998) to transform their deficit so that it was no longer a major issue in their lives, leaving them free to contribute to life in a positive way. This is because the 16 hearing impaired people, who volunteered for this ground-breaking study, had, to a greater or lesser extent, been able to chart their own course in life and had not allowed themselves to be dictated to by traditional British norms which unfortunately still too often frown on disabled people taking responsibility for their own lives and becoming autonomous and contributing members of society.

A gap in our understanding

Looking at the broader field of social policy, despite a burgeoning quantity of research on disability, marriage and family life, studies of marriage and disability are still rare (Parker, 1993). There is, however, some reference to the experience of married people (Blaxter, 1976) as well as personal accounts (Kisor, 1990).

The dearth of research in this area may be related to the interests and foci of different academic disciplines. The social policy literature has attempted to map the impact of various disabilities on people, specifically deprivations caused by society (Sainsbury, 1986). Only after the deprivations have been made explicit is it then possible to begin to look at their impact on relationships, specifically the psychosocial dimension.

The feminist literature has also tended to ignore the relational processes within families by focusing on women's caring role (Lewis and Meredith, 1988). Although a broader and more varied focus is explored by Doucet (1995), so far only a limited interest has been shown in couples or in seeing this caring process as a mutual endeavour.

Psychologists, sociologists, social psychologists and child health experts have been interested in families and disability, but more from the perspective of the welfare of the children rather than their parents (Thurman, 1985). However, there have been exceptions, for example in social policy (Baldwin, 1985), social psychology (Quine and Pahl, 1985) and in applied family and child studies (Earhart and Sporakowski, 1984).

The study of the implications of hearing impairment on the family might also be thought of concern to the Church. In the ageing population, three-quarters of the 7.5 million adults in the UK judged to have an acquired hearing loss, are over 60 years of age. However, in the 150 page report published by the Social Policy Committee of the Board of Social Responsibility of the Church of England, there is no mention of hearing loss (Ageing, 1990).

Contemporary British research in the field of deafness itself is still in its infancy (Jones, Kyle and Wood, 1987; Beattie, 1981). Much of what has been done has focused on prelingually profoundly deaf people (Sainsbury, 1986). While this group now has a higher profile, people with acquired hearing loss continue to be neglected and notoriously to suffer from long-term identity confusion caused by not knowing where they belong (Harvey, 1989; Thomas, 1984).

This is all the more puzzling as the number of people with acquired hearing loss greatly outstrips the number of people who are prelingually deaf. For example in Great Britain, for every one prelingually deaf person, there are approximately 150 people who have acquired hearing loss. This in depth study includes only one prelingually deaf person and 15 people with acquired hearing loss. The ratio was considered appropriate in view of the neglect of the larger group of people with late onset deafness.

Studying an old problem in a new way

A working hypothesis was developed suggesting that couples who contained a hearing impairment within their relationship needed to assess how it was affecting the quality of couple and family relational processes. Furthermore, if this was not done regularly throughout the life-cycle, it was predicted that familial processes would deteriorate in quality or not develop appropriately. Two crucial medical factors influencing this working hypothesis were the degree of hearing impairment experienced and the age of onset.

For this hypothesis to be tested, a method had to be found whereby it would be possible to study hearing loss within the marital relationship. This is because while working previously with couples as a social worker and marriage guidance (RELATE) counsellor, I learned what a powerful force for health or illness the marital interaction of a couple could be and could become. The importance of this dimension was reinforced by additional course work and supervision received at the Tavistock Institute of Marital Studies. This interest in interviewing couples led to the marital and family literature, and family sociology specifically work by Elizabeth Bott. As her study of *Family and Social Networks* most nearly approached the type of research required, it was adopted with certain adaptations (Bott, 1957). In using her approach along with other theoretical material, I have been able to produce a qualitative/anthropological study which illuminates the interaction between people's psychosocial experiences and the medical and audiological nature of hearing impairment.

The small numbers in the Bott study and the intensive interviewing involved provided an opportunity to establish the psychosocial factors which can modify or exacerbate the impact of hearing impairment on relationships. Such knowledge is intended to help clinicians (Corker, 1994) and researchers to have a deeper picture of the lives of hearing impaired people that incorporates both positive and negative dimensions; and helps to lessen the likelihood that they will project their own negative fantasies on to their patients, clients and respondents (Romano, 1984).

While it is not possible in this study to replicate the interdisciplinary team approach of Bott, it was simulated to a certain extent. A range of skills was employed including those derived from marriage counselling and social work as well as personal experience of hearing impairment to identify the psychological as well as the social and policy dimensions of hearing impairment in couple relationships. As Bott's focus was on so-called normal families, it gave no help in finding out how disability, specifically deafness of a partner in tandem with that of the researcher, would affect the developing methodology. The literature provides a number of examples where deaf researchers were used, the most helpful of which were the remarks of deafened researcher, Peter Wood:

> Overall the presence of a deafened researcher is I believe not only beneficial but probably essential. In dealing with acquired hearing loss where the implications are to a large extent subjective and psychological ... (Jones, Kyle and Wood, 1987: 202)

From experience of having taken part in 150 intensive interviews with hearing impaired people while being impaired myself, I support these views. However, there are also other important factors which help enhance the effectiveness of a hearing impaired researcher, including a reliable grasp of lip-reading, previous interviewing skill, and an ability to notice and accurately interpret visual cues. It is also especially helpful to nurture an inner dialogue between the part of oneself which identifies with being hearing impaired and the part which identifies with being hearing to help achieve a balanced perspective.

The couple relationship is in fact the most complex of all human relationships. Because of this, it is important to explore at this point a few of the understandings which have been developed over the years in an attempt to explain its nature.

Ways of looking at marriage

Marriage and family may be seen as being in transition from institution to companionship (Mace, 1981). When closely observed, these two aspects of marriage are in interplay with each other in some form of coexistence (Mansfield and Collard, 1988). Factors such as the social emancipation of women, the emphasis on personal fulfilment, and the disassociation of sex from procreation through contraception, led to a tendency to see marriage as a source of emotional fulfilment as well as a social duty. Consequently, couples appear to stay together because of a combination of external constraints coming from the public sphere and a relational component sometimes referred to as 'internal cohesion' found in the private sphere.

A sociological perspective

If sufficient internal cohesion is the hallmark of today's flourishing marriage, it is important to look more deeply at the elements which contribute to its development. For many years the functionalist approach (Parsons and Bales, 1955) dominated sociological thinking about marriage. They focused on sex-role divisions within marriage, and are best known for their distinction between the 'instrumental' role of the husband and the 'expressive role' of the wife. This theory, however, does not adequately explain the changes taking place today in marriage and has failed to see the multi-faceted patterns of sex-role divisions in marriage and how roles, expectations, and relationships of husband and wife have been influenced by social change.

There is a contrasting approach which emphasizes conflict and change in opposition to consensus and stability. Although there is a variety of slightly differing schools of thought within this approach, they all recognize three fundamental concepts: conflict, bargaining and power. The basic assumption is that without some means of avoidance or resolution, partners in a marriage will inevitably conflict with each other. Although acknowledgement of conflict is very important, there is much in the literature to suggest that this is not the foundation on which to build a whole theory of marriage.

Therefore, a third approach is required for a deeper understanding of 'internal cohesion'. This concept's basic assumptions can best be described as falling in to the symbolic-interactionalist school. There are three basic tenets of this approach which are relevant to this study. First, one cannot understand social behaviour without understanding an individual's own interpretation of objects, situations or the actions of others (Blumer, 1962). Thus marriage processes cannot be understood without an examination of how the participants themselves define what is taking place (Berger and Kellner, 1964). Secondly, symbolic interactionism holds that although the behaviour of husbands and wives is constrained by the norms or expectations of society, it is not determined by them. It believes both that individuals interpret norms and expectations differently, and that all couples have the opportunity to make choices about their marital roles, goals and modes of operation. It is through the interaction of husband and wife that the special character and nature of each marriage emerges, as each person influences and reacts to the behaviour and attitudes of the other. Thirdly, implicit in the above, marriage is seen as a process, as a relationship which can develop or change as the couple continue to act and react to each other and to events and individuals in their external world.

The family therapist's view

By exploring the term, 'process', it is possible to acquire a fuller understanding of the term 'internal cohesion'. Satir (1972) suggests that the initial cohesive force in our Western culture is 'love', but that love alone can not sustain all the demands of married life. This is partly because there are so many unrealistic mistaken ideas about love such as, love is 'sameness' or absence of conflict, and partly because there is another ingredient altogether which may be called 'the process' in the marriage. She describes this 'process' as being the way a couple work at nurturing their loving feelings; a couple's 'process' contains many complex dimensions. It can be revealed in such things as the quality of the couple's sex life and communication, their ability to negotiate decisions and delegate tasks, their constructive management of conflict. When this 'process' is highly developed, internal cohesion is also high.

The systems perspective, another related approach, incorporates an understanding of the processes described above. Galvin and Brommel (1991) list eight assumptions which outline this approach. Four of the fundamental assumptions will be discussed here. First, in order to understand individuals fully, their functioning must be understood within the primary system of the family. Secondly, in committed relationships, cause and effect become interchangeable over time. Therefore, to understand what is happening, the present interaction rather than the past is the primary focus. Thirdly, human behaviour is seen as the result of many variables interacting together rather than the result of one cause. This shifts the focus from individual members' behaviour to the family as a whole with its interdependent relationships. This means that family problems of any type must be viewed on many levels thus dismissing simplistic approaches. Lastly, the whole is greater than the sum of its parts whether those parts are individuals or sub-systems. Viewing the family as a system, highlights the importance of the need for accurate communication between parts of the system.

While discussions of systems and 'process' are helpful in establishing a family therapeutic theoretical foundation for the study, the question still remains, 'What determines a couple's process?' A way forward with this question is to acquire some understanding of how the unconscious works within the marital relationship.

The lens of the marital therapist

Mattinson and Sinclair (1981) suggest that there are two ways which help them to understand couples' interaction on an unconscious level. The first is John Bowlby's theory of 'attachment and loss' (1969), and is predominately a theory of individual personality. The second is the theory of marital interaction as developed at the Tavistock Institute of Marital Studies (TIMS) in its clinical work with couples.

Briefly, Bowlby believes that understanding the responses of children to the separation or loss of their mother figure is a reflection of the bond that ties them to her in the first place; for example, when young children are separated from their usual caregiver, they go through stages where they protest vigorously, despair of recovering her, and finally lose interest and become emotionally detached. He defines attachment behaviour as 'seeking and maintaining proximity to another individual' (1969).

Bowlby's theory informs our understanding of some of the feelings and stress which the loss of hearing could precipitate. It was hypothesized that attachment behaviour within a couple's relationship would become more pronounced and altered where one partner has a hearing impairment. There may be echoes of earlier developmental stages as testing goes on to see if the new vulnerability can be absorbed within the framework of the existing relationship. Such behaviour as clinging, dependency, compulsive independence, and doubting may set up a vicious circle which upsets the couple's established equilibrium. If the relationship is to survive in a healthy way, a new equilibrium needs to be found based upon a reassessment of the needs of both partners.

Another psychological perspective on marriage is offered by marital interaction theory. This theory suggests that marriage is more than Bowlby's 'finding a suitable object of attachment'. TIMS puts forward two other psychological purposes for marriage: one is concerned with psychological development and the other is concerned with the avoidance of psychological pain (Mattinson and Sinclair, 1981).

From the developmental point of view, the opportunity to reattach and therefore, to be in touch with feelings associated with attachment holds the promise of being able to make better what was felt to be wrong in the past, and to make partnership more satisfying than was dimly remembered from childhood. The likelihood of being able to do this is heightened by the unique combination of responsibilities of family life, and the opportunity to behave childishly within the intimacy of a sexual relationship.

Furthermore, the partners may choose each other as complements to express what they cannot express for themselves. Some of these different characteristics may be valued, and others may be feared; but if they can be handled within the current situation, and experienced as less destructive than previously, healing takes place. It is thus possible to understand C.G. Jung's vision (1925) of marriage as an 'emotional container'. Just as a young child needs to be contained and given a 'home base', so too may adults develop more of their fullness of nature if provided with an emotional container.

How then may our understanding of marital interaction theory be applied to a marriage when one partner is hearing impaired? It is likely that defences will develop to ward off the reality of the deafness and its implications. Mattinson and Sinclair define 'defences' as the techniques the ego uses when the conscious mind is under greater strain than it can bear (1981). Such strain may be caused by pain, anxiety or conflict. The whole notion of 'defences' owes more to Freud and classical psychoanalysts than to Bowlby. Freud suggests that the defences of repression, denial and splitting of the ego are often traced to experiences of loss. This could apply to the loss of hearing.

Of these three defences, 'splitting' is particularly important in our discussion of deafness and marriage as it may contribute to the 'denial' of the problem. The defence of 'splitting' may be described as a mechanism whereby, when a person has conflicting feelings about something such as a partner's deafness, either the positive or the negative feelings drop into the unconscious. This is believed to occur when the hearing partner has not fully accepted their partner's deafness. The hearing impaired partner then receives the unconscious message that they must keep anything negative connected with their hearing loss outside the marriage boundaries and true integration does not take place. An example of this process will be discussed in Chapter 4.

Thus marriage, and more specifically marriage where one partner is hearing impaired, may be viewed from a number of different theoretical perspectives. These perspectives are then made useful in the way in which they inform not only the interviewing in the study, but also the reader of this book. Appendices A and B contain more information about the actual people who took part in this study. Most details have been changed to protect the confidentiality of the study participants.

Summary

Discussion in this chapter is about the use of an anthropological/ethnographic approach when examining the impact of hearing impairment on family life. Although the survey approach has previously been useful in conveying many of the problems experienced by hearing impaired people, ethnography is a more satisfactory approach because it is better able to reveal the multi-faceted aspect of the problem.

Also discussed was the importance of maintaining a disciplined 'dual focus' when interviewing hearing impaired people about their lives. By focusing on both 'deafness' and 'family', both positive and negative aspects of the problem are revealed resulting in the emergence of a more balanced picture of hearing impaired people.

Hearing impaired researchers were perceived as being essential in this process provided they enter the field well prepared and supported. Although it might be argued that this would hold true for the execution of any successful research and that stress is an inevitable part of the research process, hearing impaired researchers are likely to experience additional problems. If some of these problems are discussed before entering the field, the work is more likely to be executed with competence.

A number of perspectives from different fields are outlined as being useful. The systems approach used in family therapy, psychoanalytic insights from marital therapy, symbolic interactions from sociology, and the family life-cycle from developmental psychology all facilitate insight. The latter was particularly useful when analysing some of the remarks of the 28 children covered by the study.

Lastly the point is made that this study is well founded despite/because of its small size in that the sample is representative of a very large range of people medically and developmentally. Hearing impaired people in every stage in the life-cycle are included. The people came from a wide range in terms of background and social factors, for example class, education, ethnicity and religion which makes for more interesting comparisons and succeeds in breaking a way from the negative stereotype of the depressed isolated and helpless hearing impaired person of past studies. The discussion now moves to consider the dual focus of the study.

Plan of the book

Following the introductory chapter, Chapters 2 and 3 establish the context of the book from the medical/audiological and the psychosocial perspectives. Chapters, 4, 5 and 6 explore the impact of hearing loss on couples and families. Chapter 4 examines how hearing loss may affect couples when they are initiating serious relationships. Chapter 5 discusses the impact of hearing loss on more established couple relationships, and Chapter 6 explores the evolution of these relationships. Chapter 7 looks at the impact on hearing children when one of their parents has a hearing loss and the other hears normally. Chapters 8, 9 and 10 focus on the impact of hearing loss on social networks. Chapters 8 and 9 examine how hearing loss makes an impact on kinship and wider networks respectively. Chapter 10 concludes this section with an exploration of the double loss of hearing and a marital partner. Chapter 11 explores provisions for people with acquired hearing loss in the UK, and Chapters 12 and 13 summarize the conclusions of the study, offering charts as well as verbal text and lastly leading to suggestions for ways forward.

CHAPTER 2

Hearing loss

The major concerns of this book are the psychosocial consequences of acquired hearing loss. Before exploring them, it is necessary to have a background understanding of the relevant medical and audiological factors. This chapter examines the nature of acquired hearing loss and makes an important distinction between prelingual deafness and acquired hearing loss. It continues by considering the two factors believed to have the most impact on adjustment: the time of onset and the degree of loss. Then follows a discussion of other salient factors such as types of hearing loss, aetiology, rapidity, and the nature of residual hearing. The discussion then shifts to exploring the psychosocial implications of acquired hearing loss. The literature is reviewed specifically in connection with mental health issues, personal identity and social networks, group identity, bereavement stages, stress, and stigma. We begin with a definition of acquired hearing loss.

Medical and audiological factors

Broadly speaking, acquired and/or late onset deafness is hearing impairment which occurs later in life. 'Later', however, has no standard definition. Furth (1973) defines 'late' onset deafness as developing as early as the years of language acquisition. Others see it as occurring at or later than puberty (Jones, Kyle and Wood, 1987). The second definition suffices in this book.

Traditionally, clinicians have seen the time of onset and the degree of deafness as the most significant factor in predicting the level of adjustment (Cowrie and Douglas-Cowrie, 1987).

Other significant descriptive factors are prevalence, type of loss, rapidity and the nature of the residual hearing. The discussion will begin with prevalence so as to provide a statistical context and some hard evidence.

Prevalence

Hearing impaired people do not form a homogeneous group. They differ in many ways. Research suggests that 17 per cent of the adult population in Great Britain have a hearing loss of 25 decibels or more (Royal National Institute for the Deaf Research Group, 1990). This population may be further subdivided between prelingually deaf people and those with an acquired hearing loss. It has been estimated that there are 25,000 profoundly prelingually deaf people of all ages living in Great Britain. In contrast, there are approximately ten million people with acquired hearing loss in the UK (Jones, Kyle and Wood, 1987), the majority of whom are over the age of 60. At the other end of the age range, the number of children born with some degrees of deafness is approximately three in every 1000 births. In addition to this, many children experience fluctuating hearing problems associated with middle ear infection('glue ear') during childhood.

Previous researchers sometimes confused prelingually deaf individuals with the much larger population of people with late onset deafness. Since 11 out of the 16 hearing impaired people interviewed in this study acquired their hearing losses after the age of 25, the primary focus here will be those with acquired hearing loss.

Prevalence may also be measured by considering communication strategies used. The number of people with National Health Service hearing aids is now estimated as approaching two million; and at least half a million own commercial hearing aids (some of whom will also have NHS aids). Since there are four million potential hearing aid users in the UK, there is still a considerable gap between the number who have hearing aids and the number who would be likely to benefit from them. Statistics on NHS provision indicate that there is higher uptake of hearing aids among the more severely affected end of the potential population (RNID Research Group, 1990). Researchers estimate that 70–80 thousand people communicate manually in the UK (Sainsbury, 1986). There are no statistics available concerning the number of people who use lip-reading as a communication strategy.

Time of onset

Time of onset is significant because individuals whose hearing loss occurs before language has developed will have very different life experiences and present themselves in a much different manner from those whose hearing loss has occurred subsequently in childhood, adolescence, maturity or old age (Heller, Flohr and Zegan, 1987). It is also suggested that both an individual's current age and the age of onset will give an indication of the meaning of hearing loss to the individual. If the loss is first suffered at a stage of life when it was felt to be untimely or exceptional, it is experienced as more threatening than the same disorder (for example presbycusis) encountered at a later stage such as between the ages of 60 and 70. At this time it is seen as expected and part of the ageing process (Humphrey, Gilhome-Herbst and Faurqi, 1981).

The degree of deafness

The degree of deafness is also seen to be important as it indicates how well a person can understand human speech. Hearing loss is usually measured in terms of the quietest sounds a person can hear using a decibel scale and a pure tones test. There are various ways of describing what a given loss means in practice.

The following is based on the American Committee on Conservation of Hearing:

26–40 dB	mild-Difficulty only with faint speech
41–55 dB	moderate-Frequent difficulty with normal speech
56–70 dB	moderate-Frequent difficulty with loud speech
71–90 dB	severe-Understand only shouted or amplified speech over 90 dB
>90 dB	profound-Usually cannot understand even amplified speech

These categories are to be seen as coarse descriptions of very complex issues (Cowrie and Douglas-Cowrie, 1987). They may also be used to understand roughly the range of loss found in the 16 hearing impaired people in the study. It is, however, very important not to use these classifications to draw any fixed conclusions since two individuals with the same degree and patterning of hearing loss may differ markedly in actual speech discrimination ability, in cultural identification, and overall adjustment. Nevertheless, some very rough guidelines are used. Assuming that the loss is equal for both ears, with a mild loss, the person begins to strain to hear, may raise the volume of the television a bit and occasionally, ask for repetition and give wrong answers. If the person has a moderate loss, there is a need for frequent repetition, much louder volume of television, frequent wrong answers and misunderstood words in group conversations, and noticeable fatigue from listening intently. A severe loss is evident to everyone and usually requires a hearing aid. The person with a profound loss hears only very loud sounds if anything.

From the degree of loss, the focus moves to the type of hearing loss.

Two types of hearing loss

There are two main types of hearing loss: conductive and sensorineural. Anything which inhibits the passage of sound from its source to the inner ear results in a conductive loss. Generally a conductive loss is not considered as serious as other types because it can be treated medically and surgically. However, positive medical interventions may occasionally precipitate psychological or marital difficulties (Dueck, 1984). This is because it is likely that a certain relational equilibrium was reached before the operation, and a new one will have to be re-established afterwards. Discussion of specific marital issues connected with adjustment to hearing loss is found in Chapter 5.

One of the most common types of conductive hearing loss to be treated surgically is otosclerosis. This is an inherited condition and genetic counselling is recommended for family members. It affects the bony capsule surrounding the inner ear. As the disease gradually destroys the healthy bone, a soft highly vascular bone develops, resulting in the stapes (stirrup bone) becoming stuck in the oval window. In this position the stapes can no longer vibrate and a conductive hearing loss occurs. Otosclerosis and other conductive losses respond well to the use of a hearing aid which means that if the inner ear is normal, there is usually little difficulty with distortion.

Conversely, the use of hearing aids and other assisting devices providing mere amplification or refinement of sound, are insufficient to improve a sensorineural loss because of the distortion which takes place. With the exception of the cochlear implant operation, there is still no effective medical or surgical treatment which may be offered to people with senorineural loss. It is for this reason that learning the skill of lip-reading is an essential rehabilitation strategy.

Thus, the seriousness of this type of hearing loss results from its nearly imperceptible onset and insidious progress which medical intervention at this time is unable to correct. However, this fact has also challenged researchers; and, as a result of continual experiments with birds and rats, insights into the nature and regeneration of sensory hair cells are emerging (Rubel, 1994).

The exact aetiology of sensorineural hearing loss is varied and complex. For example hearing impairment may be caused by noise, experience of ototoxic drugs, the ageing process, genetic inheritance, and infections. It is the high fever caused by the latter, for example in scarlet fever, diphtheria and meningitis, which is likely to damage the hair cells. Without question, however, the commonest cause of a sensorineural hearing impairment is the 'wear and tear' of old age. This occurrence causes the loss of acuity in the mechanisms of the inner ear resulting in a condition which resembles sensorineural loss generally. This type of hearing loss is bilateral, symmetrical and is known as presbycusis. It is now believed to have a major genetic component.

A puzzling question is why hearing loss is more pronounced in some people(s) than in others. It is thought that the rapidity and degree of impairment may be influenced by the specific lifetime of the ear particularly by exposure to noise. Evidence found by Rosen suggests that members of primitive societies where there is little noise pollution, have sharper hearing than their counterparts in industrial societies (Rosen el al., 1982).

A similar parallel may be found in understanding why older women experience less hearing loss than older men. Although this fact may be changing along with women's roles generally, in the past they have encountered less superfluous noise in their lives since excessive noise levels in the home are usually easier to control than outside. Alternatively, the most significant factor here could be the absence of stress. Rosen found evidence for this also in his studies of elderly members of primitive tribes. They were found to have less heart disease as well as more acute hearing (1982).

Other factors

There are other audiological factors to be considered when assessing the impact of sensorineural hearing impairment on adjustment. First, there is the rapidity of hearing loss. Reactions to hearing impairment vary according to whether its onset is sudden or gradual. When people are suddenly deafened, personal accounts suggest there are likely to be sharp pangs of grief in contrast to a more diffuse sense of mourning that accompanies a gradual loss (Mulrooney, 1973).

This question of the rapidity of loss may also explain why there is often some ambiguity in respondents' reported time of onset, for example, hearing losses are often experienced gradually and consequently long periods of time elapse before they are noticed and considered problematic.

Another factor is the specific nature of the residual hearing, often determined by a number of sub-factors such as aetiology, rapidity and type of hearing loss. For example, some people may have residual hearing in the higher frequencies, the lower frequencies, or both. Depending on the frequencies and patterning of the remaining hearing, it is usually possible to provide a hearing aid for sounds in the speech range; or failing this, for grosser environmental sounds. In recent years, the cochlear implant operation has provided deafened people with a means of hearing some of these sounds.

There are a number of complications or side effects associated with residual hearing. Tinnitus, recruitment and vertigo are the most common. Tinnitus is a condition which produces unremitting or recurrent ringing in the ears of greater or lesser intensity with no apparent outside stimulus. While it is most often associated with sensorineural loss, it has been known to accompany conductive hearing loss and normal hearing. Recent reports suggest that 50 per cent of the people who complain of a hearing loss to their doctors in the UK also complain of tinnitus. At present there is no cure although some people find masking devices, positive thought and relaxation techniques to be useful. The phenomenon of recruitment means that a relatively slight increase in the intensity of sound results in a disproportionate increase in the sensation of loudness. This may cause the dynamic range of hearing to lessen. Cases have been reported where fairly loud sounds which cause little discomfort to hearing people cause stress and pain to those with a hearing impairment. This disorder is thought to be caused by sensory cell damage. Vertigo is a complication most often associated with Menière's disease. The symptoms include repeated sudden attacks of whirling vertigo, accompanied by nausea and vomiting. These episodes may last any time from ten minutes to eight hours. Tinnitus may also accompany this condition. These specific complications have been explored since they were experienced by the people in this study.

Psychosocial implications

An acquired hearing impairment is more than likely to disrupt relationships since the ability to hear is so central to relational processes. It is evident that having a hearing impairment is not merely about the physical process of not hearing, nor is it just about the frustrations which are felt in losing access to a certain level of information and conversation. Seen from this psychosocial perspective, the problem is much deeper and more encompassing in that it strikes at the heart of all social relationships in both the private and public sphere. With limited rehabilitation and organizational support, or social awareness, people with declining hearing in the UK have had to cope with a minimum of help at work, at home and in social settings. This has been documented vividly in personal accounts by clinicians and researchers.

This chapter and the last endorse the systems perspective. People are considered as part of an overall context, not simply as individuals with a personal problem. Individuals do not exist without a context. Therefore, a communication problem such as acquired hearing loss may be seen as belonging to the individual, but also and equally belongs to the family, social networks and to the whole of society.

Mental health issues

There are implications in the systems approach for looking at the mental health of people with acquired hearing loss. Researchers and clinicians suggest that negative behavioural and emotional characteristics presented by many deaf and hard of hearing clients have emerged and are supported as a function of the interaction within and between systems. Although it is not always the case, this statement implies that the majority of mental health problems of deaf and hearing impaired people are rooted in context, not personal pathology. Harvey argues that such problems are often the result of interactions with people who have generally negative attitudes about deafness and hearing impairment, although these attitudes may be disguised as concern (1989).

Moreover, there is a tendency of personal accounts to emphasize the traumatic aspects of hearing loss (Hunt, 1944). The affected person is seen as anxious, withdrawn, suspicious, hostile and lonely. This stereotype has repeatedly been reinforced by other studies which attempt to find a link between hearing loss and psychological disturbance. Although in no way questioning the importance of these early studies, recent research has sought to question the comprehensiveness of such evidence.

In the past decade, as deafness has begun to be depathologized, more hopeful personal accounts have been written (Kisor, 1990; Glennie, 1990). These accounts show that it is possible for a hearing impaired person not only to achieve a tenable position in the hearing world, but also to be acknowledged as a public figure. In addition, the more intimate details of family life and friendship development have emerged. Alongside these autobiographical accounts, a new generation of research has attempted to overcome some of the past sampling and methodological difficulties (Thomas, 1984; Jones, Kyle and Wood, 1987).

Unfortunately, with few exceptions, previous studies have tended to reinforce the model of deafness as a pathological state. For example, Thomas discovered that 'although severe hearing loss was not associated with a very high level of psychological disturbance as in the first study, hearing impaired adults were still nearly four times more likely to be psychologically disturbed than were normal people' (1984: 125). The psychological disorders existed at the 'psychoneurotics' level and did not result in obvious abnormal behaviour.

Wax (1989) argues that such pathological labels must be viewed with suspicion since hearing impaired people are measured against mainstream 'hearing' norms and standards. A more effective paradigm is to examine psychological and mental health norms so as to perceive what constitutes appropriate cognitive, affective and behavioural standards and norms for deaf and hearing impaired people. Sussman (1986) proceeds by identifying 'overcoming skills' or key characteristics of the psychologically healthy deaf person. They include the following:

(a) positive psychological acceptance of hearing impairment;
(b) positive self-concept/self-esteem;
(c) ability to cope with negative and/or patronizing attitudes;
(d) assertiveness;
(e) ability to place speech ability in perspective;
(f) positive attitudes toward communication devices;
(g) socialization with other hearing impaired people;
(h) ability to survive 'misguidances';
(i) philosophical and unhostile sense of humour;
(j) *gemeinschafftegefuhl* (joy of life).

Although primarily developed in relation to members of the Deaf community, this list is also relevant for people with acquired hearing loss.

Personal identity and social networks

The concept of 'personal identities' is used here as a way of exploring how individual differences affect the way people with acquired hearing loss respond to the constraints felt. Erikson defines personal identity as 'the ability to express oneself as something that has continuity and sameness, and to act accordingly' (1965: 37). He sees adolescence as the major time for formulating identity (personal, sexual, occupational and ideological) in preparation for adult life. Other times of 'identity crisis' occur throughout life especially at significant transition points such as marriage, divorce, birth of children, geographical relocation, changes of occupation or status, redundancy, retirement and bereavement.

Identity disruption is most strongly felt in the specific areas of social communication and body image (Eichler, 1981). Since most people are socialized in the dominant hearing culture, the deafened person is most likely to have absorbed the view that hearing loss is a physical disability with connotations of pathology and stigma. Thus it is understandable that Levine (1960) detects trauma (an upset in psychic balance) in the response of those recently afflicted as opposed to the relatively contented outlook of those born deaf. While prelingually deaf people have in most cases developed in the company of their deaf associates, those with acquired hearing loss find themselves isolated without a congenial 'reference group' (Hyman, 1942). Hetu, Jones and Getty (1993) even suggest that the family, or the partner specifically, may then become a substitute for the deafened peron's lost 'social world'.

Group identity

The difficulties experienced by people with acquired hearing loss will be explored further after a brief look at how sociologists view 'communities' and how prelingually deaf people and their theoreticians have adapted this view.

Most sociologists are in basic agreement that communities consist of people in 'social interaction with a geographical area and having one or more additional common ties' (Hillery, 1955). It is felt that this definition, minus the geographical requirement in most instances, broadly characterizes the Deaf community. The emphasis is primarily on common characteristics, experiences, language, type of education, needs, interests, and self-identification. Another perspective sees the Deaf community also as an ethnic minority group (Sacks, 1990).

Other scholars disagree about whether or not there is a Deaf community; and if so, how unified it really is. Padden and Humphries (1988) choose to emphasize its unity by following precedent in using lower case 'deaf' when referring to the audiological condition of not hearing, and the upper case 'Deaf' when referring to a particular group of deaf people who share a language (for example, American Sign Language) and a culture. They argue that American and Canadian members inherit their sign language, use it as a primary means of communication between themselves, and hold a set of beliefs about themselves in relation to the larger society. Participation in the life of the Deaf community has been briefly described here since it is one of the 'lifestyle choices' for people who lose their hearing in adult life. 'Lifestyle' in this context is referring to the 'enduring patterns of living, loving and working in the world' (Wax, 1989: 143).

One person in the study chose the Deaf community as his lifestyle choice, but after he married his hearing wife, they became 'bicultural'.

Four possible lifestyle choices have emerged. Those who choose the Deaf community are described as maintaining a lifestyle which segregates them partially as a social minority group from the larger hearing world (Glickman, 1986). The hard of hearing, the second group, are usually 'mainstreamed' into the larger hearing world and tend to become part of the same cultural framework as most service providers. With two exceptions, this was the 'lifestyle' chosen by all the people in this study. The third group consists of deaf and hard of hearing people who are 'biculturals' and can move between the Deaf culture and mainstream society; these people tend to be bilingual and have a broad range of social skills learned in both worlds. A final group could be considered 'marginal' in that they do not fit well into either Deaf or hearing worlds. Because this group tends to be withdrawn and isolated, they are often lost to service providers unless some significant event such as hospitalization or involvement in research brings them into contact with the outside world (Wax, 1989).

Each lifestyle choice has its own potential advantages and disadvantages. For example, individuals who choose to identify strongly with the Deaf community may have a strong sense of belonging and a platform for their demands; but like members of other minority groups, they may become objects of discrimination. 'Assimilationists' is the name sometimes given to members of the second hard of hearing group. They choose to preserve an illusion of equality by 'passing' in the majority hearing culture, but may experience some sacrifice of self identity in that their hearing impairment is not always considered. Bicultural individuals who move fairly easily between the Deaf and hearing cultures have sophisticated flexible or adaptable social skills, but may experience a lack of belonging or clear sense of identity. Finally those who choose to withdraw or become isolated may experience loneliness and depression even though they may be spared considerable hearing loss related stress and embarrassment (Wax, 1989).

The assimilationists' position is the one adopted by most people with acquired hearing loss. This is because they have already established lifestyles, marriages, families, careers, leisure and social activities which they understandably wish to continue. In most instances, this lifestyle choice is possible provided assistive aids are available and used and situational limitations are accepted. However, even with a strong assimilation position, change must be acknowledged. This is illustrated in the following discussion of bereavement stages.

Bereavement stages

The acceptance of acquired hearing loss is deeply rooted in the need to acknowledge and to grieve for what has been lost. Stages from disability and bereavement theory have been borrowed to describe the journey taken by the hearing impaired individual (Kubler-Ross, 1970).

These vary, but usually include some aspects of the following: denial; anger; guilt; depression; and adaptation. Further explanation is given for understanding these stages by adding the following points: (1) the stages do not always happen in this order; (2) there is no time limitation on any one stage; (3) not everyone experiences all these stages; (4) some never experience any of these stages. However, even after some degree of personal mourning has occurred, social interaction must still be faced.

We now look at how the literature views such interactions.

Stress

Anxiety and stress reduction are a primary motivation in human behaviour (Sullivan, 1953). While agreeing with the universal nature of stress, it is posited that hearing impaired people feel more anxiety and stress because of their communication difficulties; and therefore they are likely to engage in more anxiety/stress reduction behaviours. Depending upon various factors, this behaviour may have positive or negative consequences. Before exploring these factors, let us look more closely at the nature of stress.

Stress is described as a biological and psychological reaction to threatening and unpleasant circumstances in which the individual involved feels at a disadvantage (Sarason, 1980). The biological changes referred to include increased pulse rate, high blood pressure, perspiration, headaches, constricted blood vessels, constipation and hormonal changes. Stress is seen as a normal reaction and can even be helpful at times such as when it signals danger. Like most psychological mechanisms stress is subjective, meaning that only limited generalizations may be made about its functioning, for example, stress generated in a given situation may act as a challenge to one person and stimulate fear in another.

Compared with the experience of people with acquired hearing loss, prelingually deaf people, despite and because of their greater deficit, may experience less stress than those with acquired hearing loss. Perhaps this is because they are more or less resigned to their limitations and experience serious problems of communication with non-signers as purely practical in nature to be negotiated with little emotional investment, rather like travelling in a foreign country. However, the response does appear to be variable since other members of the Deaf culture have admitted to experiencing encounters with naive hearing people as 'ego deflating' (Becker, 1980). Also if the sound of a conversation happens to be emanating out of eyesight, deaf people may not know that they are missing anything. Because the residual hearing of hearing impaired people alerts them to conversations even when the content is not understood, they are often more aware when they are missing discourse, and therefore, are vulnerable to accompanying feelings of exclusion and frustration (Harvey, 1989).

Stigma

The presence of destructive attitudes in society towards people with acquired hearing loss or late onset deafness is sometimes referred to as 'stigma'. Goffman (1963) uses this term to describe a subjective and social phenomenon experienced by people who have difficulty hearing, as well as by those with other 'discreditable traits' such as mental illness, alcoholism or physical deformity. It relates historically to the aversion to and casting off of disfigured members of society, and sees the ancient Greeks as the civilization which first made use of this practice. As a culture, they were enthusiastic about visual aids and liked to cut or burn into the body a 'sign' or 'stigma' that announced that the bearer was a slave, a criminal or a traitor. Such a person would be seen as blemished, ritually polluted and to be avoided, especially in public places. The concept of 'stigma' has often been evoked as an explanation for the difficulty hearing impaired people have in making sensible adjustments to their disability. Because they are so fearful of encountering elements of 'stigma' in their social life, people with an acquired hearing loss often prefer to be lost in the hearing world rather than identify in any way with the Deaf community by learning to lip-read, to Sign, or even to wear a hearing aid.

When considering the negative attitudes which acquired hearing loss could provoke in the people inflicted, four areas emerged: feelings of living in two worlds, difficulties resulting from disrupting taken-for-granted interactions, invisibility of the disability and the over use of the psychological defence of denial.

Summary

The discussion in this chapter gives an overview of the nature of acquired hearing impairment as it is medically and audiologically distinguished from prelingual deafness. The most crucial factors when considering adjustment and rehabilitation for those inflicted are the time of onset and the degree of loss.

People who acquire a hearing loss of any degree are in danger of maladjustment because they have lost their place and identity in society and no longer feel they belong fully in either the hearing or Deaf worlds. Finally, an understanding of the systems perspective, which takes into account both the multi-faceted and rooted in context nature of hearing loss, is seen as essential if a way forward is to be found for appropriate service provision.

The next chapter completes the 'double focus' foundation of this study and introduces the nature of intimate relationships specifically that of contemporary marriage.

CHAPTER 3

Relationships

Introduction

A recurring theme in the literature is the overwhelming importance of the ability to hear in two relational processes: sociability and intimacy. Before the impact of hearing loss can be assessed, it is important to have a deeper understanding of how these two processes operate and the specific influence of gender.

Even a modest hearing loss can gravely hamper relaxed and easy sociability. In most cases understanding and enjoyment depend not only on meaning, but also on the context and inflection of words, quick repartee, interruptions, jokes, nuances and word play. Although hearing impaired people may long to integrate and affiliate with such convivial groups, they often find themselves cut adrift feeling more and more excluded. Orlans (1985) even suggests that except for those who Sign, are excellent lip-readers, or whose hearing is completely corrected by an aid, social conversation between a deafened and hearing person is seldom both full and relaxed. Rather there are only varying degrees of effort and care, fatigue, tension, truncation and/or silence.

Jones, Kyle and Wood reveal a similarly sad picture (1987). Their study suggests that the disturbance in the ease of communication caused by a hearing impairment is likely to curtail both physical and emotional intimacy. This study provides evidence to challenge this perspective.

Here we will look at the relational processes of 'intimacy', 'sociability' and an extensive discussion of how men and women differ in their requirements of both. This is followed by a discussion of the impact of hearing loss on intimacy and the breakdown of intimacy more generally. Finally, there will be a discussion of some of the issues found in contemporary marriage today.

Intimacy

Today's popular literature is inclined to present 'intimacy' as an ideal type of highly valued relatedness (Wynne, 1988), and it has even been called an ideology in its own right (Fitzpatrick, 1988). While intimacy is frequently referred to, in fact, the research literature has barely paused to define, conceptualize, or validate its nature (Schaefer and Olson, 1981). The result is a scholarly disagreement about where 'intimacy' fits in with other relational processes, and also whether or not it is an emotional luxury incompatible with the actual lifestyles, values and predisposition's of many economic and natural groups, particularly for males. Intimacy seems often to be confused with other relational processes such as self-disclosure, attachment/caregiving, sexuality, and cohesion. Such confusion needs to be further clarified.

Intimacy defined

Some kind of conceptual picture of the nature of intimacy, relevant to contemporary marriage and partnership when one partner has an acquired hearing loss, needs to be formulated. An intimate relationship according to Olson is generally one in which individuals share intimate experiences in several areas, and there is the expectation that the experience and the relationship will persist over time. He describes seven types of intimacy: (1) emotional intimacy – experiencing a closeness of feeling; (2) social intimacy – the experience of having common friends and similarities in social networks; (3) intellectual intimacy – the experience of sharing ideas; (4) sexual intimacy, the experience of sharing affection and/or sexual activity; (5) recreational intimacy – shared experiences of interests and hobbies, mutual participation in sporting events; (6) spiritual intimacy, the experience of sharing ultimate concerns, a similar sense of meaning of life and/or religious faith; (7) aesthetic intimacy – the closeness that results from the experience of sharing beauty (1975).

Because this definition points to a wide range of shared activities, it allows for more flexibility than is sometimes attached to this term. In reviewing other definitions, some emphasize the experiences while others emphasize the relationship. In Sternberg's work (1986) on the concept of 'experienced love', three components emerge: intimacy, passion and commitment. He describes the intimacy component as largely, but not exclusively as the emotional investment in the relationship. He calls it the 'warm' component in that it evokes feelings of closeness, bondedness and connectedness. It makes it possible to trust others, and to confide one's deepest fears, hopes and dreams. Although understanding of the intimacy concept varies, most researchers have agreed to perceive it as the emotional component of a loving relationship although this is rarely explicitly stated. Instead, words like warmth, sharing and acceptance are used to describe the nature of intimacy. It may even be inferred that experiences of intimacy set in motion cycles of affirmative exchanges which may lead to mutual growth and development (Dominian, 1975). The literature also cautions that although experiences of intimacy may seem all encompassing at the time, their actual content and meaning may be much more limited. It is argued that intimacy within an enduring relationship is a process which occurs over time, and is never complete (Schaeffer and Olson, 1981). This implies that there is usually some aspect of 'relating' that needs attention.

Sociability

The concept of sociability describes a set of relationships in which men are likely to be involved. Here enjoyment is arranged around specific tasks and activities. This form of sociability tends to emphasize doing things 'side by side' in group settings rather than relating in dyads; and the relationships tend to be context bound rather than free floating. Relationships formed in this manner are relatively shallow in that personal worries and other matters of consequence to the self are rarely discussed. The bantering, kidding and needling which occurs on such occasions reinforces the moratorium on self-disclosure (Allan, 1989). The literature suggests that men tend rarely to disclose their feelings unless they wish to gain advice, information or

a knowledgeable opinion. Therefore, their first priority is often problem-solving which may fit in with their task orientation to life.
Wynne argues that this is actually a realistic relational process strategy (1988). He notes that some relationships are overwhelmed by
trappings of intimacy, and consequently neglect the less glamorous
relational processes such as problem resolution and attachment/care
giving. However, men's refusal to share themselves more openly with
their wives may have a paternalistic component. For example, the
husband imagines that his wife couldn't understand or solve the
problem that is worrying him, so prefers to protect his wife rather
than share it, when in fact he may be protecting his own image
(Komarovsky, 1962).

A marital paradox

Thus scholars suggest that husbands (with their inclination towards
sociability) and wives (with their preference for intimacy) often
approach each other from worlds within which they are likely to
have developed very different sets of assumptions about the purpose
of talking. Men are often likely to ignore these differences, while
women are more aware resulting in their attempts to bridge the gap.
Mansfield and Collard argue that here is a paradox of modern
marriage (1988). On the one hand, there is the common expectation
that the roles of the modern spouse are symmetrical and a kind of
symbiotic fusion takes place, whereas the reality demonstrates that it
is the capacity to recognize and integrate these differences between
the two widely contrasting gender worlds of verbal and actual experience which is the true challenge of marriage today.

Hearing loss and intimacy

The implications of the research on intimacy for this book suggest
that a person's hearing loss, regardless of severity, should never be
seen as the prime or only factor precipitating the breakdown of a
marriage or of intimate relationships. Other salient factors discussed
have been class, gender and mental health. Undoubtedly, however,
hearing loss will dramatically curtail more masculine styles of relating such as sociability. Criswell (1979) suggests that acquired hearing
loss has a more devastating effect on men than on women. This may
be related to men's socialization in a dominant group as their 'given

superiority' makes it more difficult for them to handle their own vulnerability, especially when it deprives them of the conversational control to which they are accustomed.

Differing socialization patterns also mean that men and women are likely to talk about their hearing loss in different ways. Jones, Kyle and Wood (1987) find that women are more likely to express frustration about their loss while men are more likely to joke about it.

Returning to Wynne's scheme for relational processes, although 'intimacy' is perceived as rare, his other relational processes are fundamental and will be used in Chapters 5 and 6 to analyse the study findings concerning continuing relationships. A brief introduction to them is given here.

A: The epigenetic principle

Wynne (1988) explains that this concept refers to events of 'becoming' ('genesis') that built 'upon' ('pi') the immediately preceding events. He sees this principle as one which is generally accepted among scientists and sets limits on the range of variability, but that within this range, random variation takes place. Wynne's Epigenetic Schema develops as follows:

1. Attachment and caregiving

Our understanding of attachment/caregiving processes is largely drawn from Bowlby. His definition is derived from his observations of young children when they were separated from or lost their mother. Bowlby believes that attachment behaviour is biologically based and may be found in the primates of all species, and is therefore the prototype of all parent–child relatedness. He suggests that attachment in adults is an expression of the same emotional system as that in children (1975).

2. Communication

At a very general level, communication is defined as a symbolic and transactional process, that is the process of creating and sharing meanings. It is symbolic in that words are used as symbols to transmit messages. It also includes the whole range of nonviable behaviours, for example facial expressions, eye contact, gestures, movement, postures, appearance and special distance (Galvin and Brommel, 1991).

3. Joint problem-solving

When the above relational tasks have been mastered to a certain degree, satisfactory problem-solving is more likely to develop. This process emphasizes the need for shared engagement in day-to-day tasks, interests and recreational activities. When transitions or crises occur during the family life-cycle, the joint problem-solving skills are 'in place', and may be drawn upon to cope with these extra stressful times. If this effort is not made, problem-solving becomes ineffective, indecisive and disorganized resulting in dysfunctional families at times of transitions.

4 (a) Mutuality or the shaping of couple relationships

Wynne (1988) uses the term 'mutuality' to refer to the partners' shared commitment to one another to shape their relationship as the life-cycle enfolds. The relational process of 'mutuality' begins with the recognition of difficulties that cannot be resolved within the framework of prior forms of relatedness such as problem-solving; and involves renegotiating and sometimes transformation to new patterns of relating. This means that there may be an expansion, a narrowing, or an ending of this relational system altogether.

Because 'mutuality' involves a commitment to an active shaping of the partnership, as opposed to a passive acceptance of it, the precise processes involved with reference to this study need to be investigated further.

Evidence from the marital therapy field suggests that a dilemma of all enduring relationships where there are differences is not only the establishment of some form of intimate experience, but also its management within the partnership. This is acknowledged in Askham's work on 'identity' and 'stability' in marriage (1984). Clulow and Mattinson describe the problem in the following way:

> couples are engaged in a kind of dance, moving towards each other and then drawing apart constantly searching for a comfortable balance in their relation-ships. Frequently the balance is no sooner found than upset again. (1989: 100)

Thus personality types and personal preferences and experiences are another dimension in the management of the appropriate distance required for intimacy. The literature also infers that the ever shifting balance or amount of intimacy (defined here as closeness, bonded-ness or connectedness), for one couple may be different for another. It is argued that it is only through experience that trust is built up, along with the feeling that it is safe to put oneself in the hands of another. Clinicians suggest that a characteristic of an adequate marriage is the ability of its partners to strike a balance between over and under engagement. Traditionally employment is one of the main areas of life which enable a married couple to achieve struc-tured distance from each other (Mattinson, 1988).

The management of distance and intimacy in enduring relation-ships is a delicate and continuous process which is continuing. Some-times an 'end' is required to the process altogether and breakdowns may occur as will be seen in the next section.

4 (b) Mutuality: breakdown of intimacy

While class, gender and mental health are factors which influence the capacity to form intimate relationships, there are other factors involved in the complete breakdown of intimacy through death and divorce.

The death of a spouse is usually harder on the husband than on the wife. Although the wife may suffer more economically, husbands are more likely to become socially isolated as a result of becoming widow-ers. Reasons for this are threefold. First, the mother is usually the one who brings the family together. Without her presence, the family may see the father less. Secondly, women are seen to have more mutuality and intimacy in their own friendships, which make it easier to adjust to widowhood. Thirdly, because traditionally men rely only on their wives as confidantes, when the wife is gone, they have no one with whom to share their feelings (Strain and Chappell, 1982). The widow and widower in this book are discussed in Chapter 10.

Likewise a similar experience may take place for men after divorce (Clulow and Vincent, 1987). Because of men's traditional dependence on their wives as confidentes, a wife's departure may not only close down the social network which she has created and main-tained, it may also remove the only confidante the husband has. Nevertheless, when a marriage ends, it is likely that each partner has stopped listening to the other and intimacy may have been replaced by power struggles (1987). One-fifth of the people who participated in the study were divorced.

4 (c) Mutuality: leisure patterns

For some people there is a clear block in their lives called 'work' which has negative or positive connotations in terms of enjoyment; and there is a clear block of time that may be termed 'leisure' within which enjoyment may be pursued in various ways. Rapoport and Rapoport (1975) argue that this view is too simplistic. They suggest the situation is more ambiguous in that there are degrees of flexibility not only in the introduction of pleasurable activities in to work, but in the dispersion of work into other situations.

Mutuality in all its forms is discussed in Chapter 6. The focus now shifts to a second family schema used for the purposes of analysis in this study.

B: The Circumplex Model of Marital and Family Systems

Another way of examining specific dimensions in family life has been developed by Olson, Sprenkel and Russell (1979) and is called the Circumplex Model of Marital and Family Systems.

This model includes three dimensions: cohesion, adaptability and a facilitating communication. It is possible to view a family's cohesion and adaptability on the intersecting lines of an axis. Communication, on the other hand, is the dimension that facilitates a specific family's movement along the cohesion and adaptability spectra.

For example, in families with extremely high cohesion, the measure of how close to each other family members feel emotionally, is often referred to as 'enmeshed'. This means they are involved to the point where the experience of family members allows for little self fulfilment or autonomy. In examining the dimension of cohesion on a spectrum, 'disengaged' families are at one end and 'enmeshed' families are at the other end. Communication between members helps to develop, change, or maintain the patterns of cohesion.

The other primary dimension, adaptability, may be described as 'the ability of a marital/family system to change its power structure, role relationships, and relationship rules in response to situation and developmental stress'. As a dimension, it bears a strong resemblance to aspects of the relational process of mutuality. It operates under the assumption that family systems constantly restructure themselves as they pass through the predictable developmental stages illustrated in Chapter 7.

Adaptability also has its own spectrum with 'rigid' families who suppress change and growth situated at one end, and 'chaotic' families who never stop changing at the other. Again it is the facilitating communication which helps to sustain, develop, or change the adaptability within family patterns. Researchers suggest that functional as opposed to dysfunctional families are likely to make good use of communication in this way.

For the purposes of analysis here, the family dimensions explored in the circumplex model will be subsumed under the Epigenetic Principle. In later chapters this schema has been used to analyse more specifically families where one partner is hearing impaired.

An overview of contemporary marriage

Recent years have seen many changes in the patterns of marriage and family life. In a relatively short period of 25 years, conventional family life has been condemned for its suffocating intimacy (Leach, 1968), denounced as a system of mystification, scapegoating and violence, and identified as a site of female subordination and exploitation. However, in spite of this onslaught of academic challenge (Segal, 1983), the family has not been abolished and continues in both traditional and altered forms. Although the institution of marriage survives, there is empirical evidence to suggest that there are 'troubles' of the type that will not disappear by labelling them social constructions (Clark and Haldane, 1990). Perhaps these 'troubles' are partly related to the disjunctions which have been created as the institution of marriage moves from being a legalistic institution to becoming more humane in its understanding of the complexities inherent in family life. This process of 'transition' has brought with it the confusion that often accompanies rapid social change (Kiely, 1984).

Regardless of change, the companionship model continues to predominate and is focused on the personal relationship between the two spouses. It involves shared activities, common interests and mutual association. There is also the built-in- expectation of intimacy, communication, sharing feelings, equity and mutual decision making. In contemplating these two marriage models, present day theorists point out that both of them contain elements of the other. For example in the companionship model, the husband is still expected to be the provider when the wife withdraws from work and they begin a family. Despite the wife's change in status, ideally the focus of marriage is still on the personal and the affective. Conversely, affective characteristics still have a place in the institutional marriage. The critical difference between the two models is that when love is present in the institutional marriage, it is welcomed; but it is not essential for survival. In the modern trend towards a companionate model, the absence of love or happiness is often grounds for its dissolution since this shift has brought with it an accompanying rise in expectations. This understanding of contemporary marriage suggests that marriage the institution now coexists with marriage the relationship.

Another central paradox of marriage today is that the relationship is thought to be important, and yet people still seek the institution. This is because marriage gives one a place within the family and a sense of continuity. Also it is a natural event, and indicates adult status and seriousness of intention.

Finally, Clulow suggests that there are four processes which are relevant to our understanding of contemporary marriage. These are the privatization of marriage, the pursuit of the egalitarian dream, the decline of absolute values and the rise of relativism, and the shifts from rights to responsibilities (1995).

Undoubtedly our understanding of the nature of marriage is in the process of change. The next sections will explore other changing aspects.

Popularity of contemporary marriage

Marriage as an institution is thriving despite setbacks and criticism. In 1995, 322,000 marriages occurred in Britain (One Plus One, 1998) making Britain and Portugal the countries which have the highest annual marriage rate in Europe (Dormor, 1990). This is 7.0 marriages per 1000 eligible population and compares with 10.0 in the USA.

Although the twentieth century has brought with it a steady increase in the popularity of the institution, this trend has slackened in the last decade in the UK. Since the early 1970s, annual first marriage rates have fallen especially for those under 25. Conversely, the average age of first marriages which reached an all-time low in 1970 has been rising (Leete, 1979). Although there has been a steady decrease in first marriages, there has also been a steady increase of second and subsequent marriages so that this group now represents 35 per cent of all marriages. The increase of second and third marriages is due to the greater ease of leaving unsatisfactory marriages following the passage of two acts: the Divorce Reform Act of 1969 which introduced the concept of 'irretrievable breakdown'; and the Matrimonial Proceedings Act of 1984 which allowed people to petition for divorce one year after marriage rather than three (Mattinson, 1988).

The exact causes of the slowing down of marriage rates are unclear, but are thought to be related to increased cohabitation, more positive attitudes towards delayed marriage in the younger generation, and economic changes which make early marriages more difficult (James and Wilson, 1986).

Contemporary trends in the couple relationship

Cohabitation

The increase in the practice of cohabitation has been linked with the present decline in the absolute numbers of marriages in Britain. Whether cohabitation may be seen as a 'trial period' leading to the marriage or a replacement of it, is debatable. Statistics show that the numbers of cohabiting couples have continued to rise so that for those married in 1987, more than one half have previously cohabited. This means that cohabitation may now be considered the norm especially for couples at the opposite ends of the social scale (Dormor, 1990). Although there is no indication that this norm is a satisfactory response to the dilemmas presented by contemporary marriage, figures recently published in 'Population Trends' (Haskey, 1992) and based on statistics from the 1989 OPCS General Household Survey suggest that the couples who live together before marriage are more than 60 per cent likely to divorce than those who do not do so. However the most recent research from the USA is starting to suggest that the increased risk of marital breakdown run by those who cohabit has decreased or is even being eliminated as cohabitation has become the usual pathway into marriage (One Plus One, 1998).

Evidence also suggests that contemporary cohabitation represents a wide range of relationships. First, the present rise in cohabitation may be connected with the higher levels of parental divorce. Having experienced first hand the failure of their parents' marriage, the children are inclined to approach formal marriage and its accompanying commitment with extreme caution. Secondly, there are stable relationships which may have evolved from earlier relationships or share accommodation. And thirdly, there are cohabiting relationships with little expectation of permanence (Burgoyne, 1985).

Divorce

The single most significant social trend in post war Britain has been the steady escalation of marital breakdown sometimes referred to as mass divorce (Clark and Haldane, 1990). The UK has, in fact, had the highest divorce rate in the European Union for many years (One Plus One, 1998). Approximately 160,000 divorces take place each year, although the proportion of divorced men and women in the adult population is only 5 per cent. Rates of divorce have been more constant since the late 1970s and Denmark has now succeeded Britain as the European country with the highest divorce figure. The implication for today's marriages is that one in three now taking place is likely to end in divorce before the 30th anniversary of the couple (Haskey, 1982).

Four factors contributing to these dramatic trends are the emancipation of women (Thornes and Collard, 1979), the demand for more intimacy within the marital relationship, the stress which this and other changes cause as marriages attempt to find a balance between the institution and the relation, and the fact that everyone is living longer meaning that being monogamous requires more restraint for a longer time (Nissel, 1987).

In fact, the psychosocial factors discussed so far suggest marriage now requires a new set of 'skills' for which couples have no preparation. Since very little education and support are offered in handling companionate marriages, divorce appears to have become a substitute solution (Dominian, 1985).

For most couples, divorce continues to bring personal pain, guilt and a sense of failure at having fallen short of the ideal of establishing something permanent. It can have adverse effects on the health of those involved, particularly men. Although conflict may have led the partners to the divorce court, the process of divorce may initiate further conflict over property, custody, access and maintenance arrangements. Some sociologists maintain that it is more helpful to see divorce as a process rather than a status: this is because it involves movement through a number of personal, emotional, material, economic and legal transitions (Burgoyne, Ormond and Richards, 1987). All the factors have the capacity to become enmeshed in a complex web. The evidence suggests that one way couples attempt to neutralize the tensions experienced is to marry again (Clark and Haldane, 1990).

Remarriage/reconstruction

Approximately one marriage in three, 120,000 each year, is now a remarriage for one or other of the partners. The most common form of remarriage is between two divorced partners. Some 50 per cent of divorced men and women remarry within five years (Clark and Haldane, 1990). Remarriage rates are about twice as high for men as for women, which is thought to be because men generally have more opportunities to meet future partners (One Plus One, 1998). Divorced men who remarry are more than one and a half times as likely to divorce as single men of the same age marrying for the first time; for divorced women, the chance is twice that of their first-married counterparts (Haskey, 1982). One interesting characteristic of remarriage is that there is a tendency for men and women to choose marriage partners who are unlike themselves in terms of age, educational background and class. In the North American literature, this practice is known as heterogamy (Clark and Haldane, 1990). Unfortunately there is not room here to discuss further contemporary family variations such as step families, one parent families, and dual earner marriages (Bernard, 1982). However, they exist and

have become a powerful force in the social construction of the term
'family' and in family social policy.

Summary

In this chapter there is a detailed discussion of contemporary
marriage and the relational processes which take place within its
boundaries.

Marriage is an immensely complex relationship which is undergoing a period of painful transition as individual couples attempt to
find an appropriate balance between the 'institutional' and the 'relational' in their lives.

In the last two chapters, the 'dual focus' of the book, namely the
nature of hearing impairment and the nature of contemporary couple
relationships, has been introduced. This has been done to give a
context to the rest of the book. In the next section, the focus shifts to
examining what can happen when a hearing and hearing impaired
person meet and begin to take each other seriously as potential partners.

PART II

Hearing Loss, Families and Social Networks

CHAPTER 4

Couples meeting

Introduction

Ten out of the 11 couples interviewed in this study were legally married. Like all contemporary couples, they had to struggle with the tensions created by the major paradox of marriage today: the relationship is thought to be all important, and yet couples continue to seek the security of the institution (Mansfield and Collard, 1988).

The family perspective in this book is that of psychosocial constructionism (Gubrium and Holstein, 1990). Attention is focused on what people say about the 'familial' in their lives, and how people construct family meaning. To speak of being 'family' is not only to use the term to describe a set of relationships, but also to convey the idea that the relationships under consideration are trusting and giving. Despite negative views which some scholars have about the family, the 'trusting and giving' referred to here is being seen in a positive light.

The 11 participating couples were divided into two groups. The first group consists of five couples where one spouse was already severely/profoundly hearing impaired at the time of their first meeting. The remaining six couples married each other with no awareness that deafness would strike one of them further into the marriage. Consequently the deaf element in the marriage was not a part of the original commitment, but was encountered after the marriage was well established.

The focus of this chapter will be on this first group of five couples where a severe/profound hearing loss is present in the midst of a heterosexual relationship. In such cases, it will undoubtedly stir up

specific issues, alongside more general themes common to all committed intimate relationships. These relationships will be discussed along
with the highly personal manner which the couples psychosocially
constructed the meaning of 'deafness as difference'. In doing so, the
couples focused on 'differences' as part of an anthropological/cultural
model rather than as a medical model (Preston, 1994). This point is
further clarified in Chapter 5 and 6 and Figure 12.1 in Chapter 12.

All couples pass through developmental stages as their relationship evolves and deepens. The five couples here passed through
three specific developmental stages: meeting and liking, getting serious, making it work.

Stage 1: Meeting and liking

Both the hearing and hearing impaired individuals need to clarify
their attitudes and feelings about the deafness factor as questions and
concerns emerge in their growing intimacy if the encounter is to be
sustained and an enduring relationship formed. In addition, their
more general attitudes to differences and problems require testing
and mutual assessment. This is because there are bound to be differences other than the deafness itself which will need to be addressed.

Conversely, if a lack of agreement is found between the potential
partners on the fundamental issue of deafness, their relationship is
likely to flounder at this early stage. If some agreement is reached,
this dialogue is the beginning of the process of finding and shaping
like-mindedness' in life more generally (Barbara, 1989).

Signs and symbols of reassurance and compliance with special needs

The hearing partner must convey reassurance to the hearing
impaired partner that 'deafness as a difference' within their relationship is seen by them as potentially manageable. Consequently, it is
not denied or seen in an unduly negative light. The use of mutually
understood symbols and/or signs conveys their reassurance. There
must also be an awareness of and compliance with 'special needs'.
For example, for some the ability to establish a quick and easy

rapport is important (Hoffmeister, 1985). Arthur, a prelingually deaf husband and student, recalled meeting his hearing wife, Gwen:

> there was never ... a serious problem ... [where] communication was concerned ... I think her range of Signs was [widening at the time we met]; she was fairly proficient. It's partly her unconscious desire to get more involved with Deaf people.

Gwen agreed:

> I found [Arthur] very easy to talk to and he seemed to be able to put up with my awful Signing ... [It] did help that there was easy communication straight away. If we had both had to struggle, perhaps it would not have gone any further.

Gwen's use of BSL and openness to further learning reassured Arthur that Gwen was sincere in her wish to have a long term involvement with Deaf people. As Harris argues:

> sign language ... use acts as a marker of willingness to conform to the core philosophical belief – that sign language is 'natural' to Deaf people. Stemming from this, my data shows that there are assertions of Deaf Clubs being 'natural sign language environments'; that BSL is many Deaf people's 'first' language and that sign language use promotes 'mental health' in Deaf People (1995: 169)

Henry, a prelingually severely deaf theological student found reassurance in his capacity to respond almost immediately to the initiatives of his future wife, Kay:

> [Kay and I] just seemed to be able to communicate with each other ... we were very open with each other, ... I think I had more hang-ups than Kay ... !

Some couples seemed to feel safer when they felt a force or person beyond themselves had brought them together. Kay talked about 'God's will' while Joe talked about 'fate'. Joe also mentioned his doctor's encouragement to attend the lip-reading class where he met his future wife, Sarah. Sarah, in turn, told how her tutor encouraged her to approach Joe:

> when we were teaching lip-reading, Joe was ... [a pupil]. It astounded me [how attractive he was] ... The teacher told us that there was a man [in the class who was tragically separated from his sons and it was him] ... I thought 'Poor man', and she told us to go and talk to him.

For Sarah, a combination of feelings and events swept her along into Joe's presence. Joe, in turn, was delighted by her attention and they discovered they shared common interests. Joe was reassured by Sarah's dedication to teaching lip-reading. He recalled:

> one evening when I got [to the lip-reading class], ... [Sarah] came up to me and said, ' How about having [the] coffee (which I had suggested earlier) with two of [my] colleagues?' I replied, 'No way, only you ... as it's enough to have to understand you, without ... try[ing] to follow the other two people as well in a café.' That was her first lesson aside from all the other lessons!

As Sarah complied with Joe's 'special needs' showing her sensitivity, Joe dared risk further involvement. Barbara, a severely deaf wife and mother, described a similar incident. She had known Ben for a number of years since they both were in the legal profession. She recounted how a severe bout of influenza helped her to resolve her doubts:

> I had 'flu ... I went [totally] deaf for three weeks – ghastly ... and I remember noticing that I could lip-read Ben even though I was totally deaf ... so in terms of verbal communication, I would say we were pretty good.

Ben's ability to be relaxed in the face of the formidable qualities of total deafness was the reassuring sign that Barbara needed. Ben confirmed her point:

> Barbara is very good at lip reading. I don't really think we have to make a great deal of effort, to be honest.

What is crucial in these examples is the ease of communication between the partners, regardless of the physical obstacle of deafness. This theme lends credibility to marital interaction theory when it supports the psychological factor or an unconscious 'couple fit' (Dicks, 1967).

The fifth couple, Julia, a textile designer, and Sam, a profoundly deaf computer programmer, was the only cohabiting couple in the study. Sam initially experienced reassurance about his deafness when Julia agreed to share his 'special need' of living a self-sufficient lifestyle. Later when they had to give up their dream for practical reasons, the commitment had transferred to their relationship.

In this way all the hearing partners communicated that 'deafness as a difference' could be managed without undue strain or sacrifice.

In fact many hearing partners in this study had encountered deafness in their past and/or were in the midst of acquiring a professional helper career in the hearing impaired field. This meant that an initial concern and interest in deafness had already taken root for them quite apart from their encounters with future spouses.

Marital researchers also suggest more generally that couple formation is aided by fortuitous events such as the individual attitudes to marriage at a particular time within a climate of events and circumstances (Mansfield and Collard, 1988). The next examples will show how these events were in operation and the resulting impact.

Fortuitous circumstances: Henry and Kay

Fortuitous circumstances were much in evidence in the meeting of Kay, a 35-year-old trained teacher who was establishing a second career in the Ministry of the Church, and her severely hearing impaired future husband. Kay recalled:

> I had been feeling that to be a woman in the Ministry who was single ... was a disadvantage, ... that if I had the authority of a husband, ... I would feel happier going into the public sort of ministry that the Church of England Ministry is, ... but ... I [wasn't] actually looking for a husband ...

She recalled her first encounter with Henry at college:

> I had no idea that Henry was deaf ... except in the beginning evening service when prayers were held and everybody gathered together ... the principal said something about sign language ... and he said it to Henry ... it stuck in my mind ...

Later when Kay and Henry happened to have coffee together, Kay asked Henry about the principal's remark and Henry explained about his deafness. Kay recalled thinking that it seemed incredible that Henry was deaf as he could communicate so well. She then decided as it did not seem to be a communication problem to Henry, why should it be for her. Kay recalled:

> [perhaps] we didn't really know each other very well, but I ... felt that [Henry] was a person who came from a similar background ... to myself as regards family, and that we had quite a lot of things in common ... we weren't totally opposite in anything except we were the opposite sex!

Henry, on the other hand, was intrigued with Kay's 'nothing unusual is happening' approach (Emerson, 1970). It reflected his own attitude and seemed more balanced than that of other women in his life. Together, Henry and Kay psychosocially constructed 'deafness as a difference' to mean an 'insignificant factor' or that everything could proceed as normal within the marriage as long as adjustments were made for 'lip-readability'.

In practice this meant that Henry had to divide himself in two: the hearing part of him was involved with his family, his studies and his work; the deaf part was to be connected with the Ministry to the Deaf which he planned to develop once he was ordained. Although not the ideal way to cope with differences, as the distancing by one partner from unconsciously perceived negative attributes of the other more often than not results in increased frustration and loneliness for that partner, Kay and Henry agreed implicitly on this method and it was maintained. Privately, Henry acknowledged:

[Kay] assumes she knows ... [what it is like to be deaf].

Although Kay talked knowledgeably about Henry's deafness and resulting pain, her actual behaviour implied that she had largely separated herself from it and there was little real room for his disability within the marriage, as revealed in her feelings of resentment when Henry didn't wear his hearing aids all the time. Although a very gifted person in many ways, a certain insecurity and lack of patience made it difficult for Kay to allow Henry the extra time and space he needed to bring his 'deafness as a difference' and accompanying feelings of isolation further into the marriage. At the same time, Henry colluded with Kay's attitude by not disclosing more of his true feelings (Willi, 1982).

This assessment was noted along with the fact that Henry and Kay, at the time of the interviews, were experiencing a very demanding period in their lives which might have given a slightly distorted picture. The following is an example of another couple who chose to manage the deafness factor in their relationship in an entirely different way, but the themes of reassurance and fortuitous circumstances are the same.

Fortuitous circumstances: Arthur and Gwen

Gwen, an infant teacher, also met her future husband, Arthur, at college:

> I had been working [and] ... I [was] on my own for about a year, saying things like, 'I'm never going to get married, ... I'm going to be a single woman with a career' ... so I certainly wasn't looking for somebody ... but [Arthur] came along, and I suppose I turned it all on its head.

Gwen felt that her interest in Deaf people had occurred long before she met Arthur. This was borne out in her commitment to learn BSL and in the preparation of a special paper on deaf/hearing integration. Arthur, like Henry, felt that here was a different sort of woman. However, the issue for Arthur with women was not the quality of sympathy, but the quality of commitment. Arthur recalled:

> It wasn't just a ... new hobby ... with Gwen, ... she took it seriously. In many ways it made an impression on me.

Gwen's affirming attitude contrasted sharply with Kay's as Arthur's did with Henry's. This may be because Arthur and Gwen were younger, and they had both found strength from involvement in Deaf culture. Henry had only just started this process, and Kay was not interested.

While Arthur's deeper feelings about his own deafness were ambivalent due to his experiences of injustice in the world, he publicly proclaimed a positive attitude towards the deafness of Deaf people generally. This position is what Harris (1995) has conceptualized as the Deaf Construction of Deafness. For the purposes of this book, Arthur and Gwen's joint perception was seen as 'deafness as a difference' being 'respectable and OK'. For Gwen there was also a sub-text. She recalled:

> when [Arthur] told me his family was Deaf, ... particularly his ... father ... and grandfather, .. I knew then that I had to start thinking seriously of what I was getting into ... I had to decide whether [hereditary deafness] was something I could cope with ... and I decided it was.

Although on the surface Gwen and Arthur presented a more united front than Kay and Henry, there were still many differences in outlook which needed to be addressed. Arthur remembered:

> I think it's more to do with [the] perception of how things should be done, [for example, ... Gwen's] perception of the world is due to having always been in a hearing environment. My parents are Deaf, and sometimes when ... [Gwen and I] argue, these perceptions are raised to the surface.

Arthur's acknowledgement of different perceptions was the first indication of what Padden and Humphries have identified as 'a different centre' often experienced by members of the Deaf community (1988).

Apart from the question of signs, symbols and compliance with mutual 'special needs', there is the question of whether or not couples are going to have children (Preston, 1994). Partners who were not parents appeared to allow more space for the integration of 'deafness of a difference' into their couple relationship as the following example illustrates.

Fortuitous circumstances: Julia and Sam

Julia met Sam at a mutual friend's house when at university. She admitted that Sam's profound deafness made little impact on her since she was caught up with her own concerns. Certainly the fact that he made nothing of it himself, and that he did not wear a hearing aid, might have made her initial insensitivity to his disability more complete. Fortuitous circumstances existed in that she found herself in an academic course which she disliked intensely and the place where she lived was cold. This contrasted with her enjoyment of being with Sam who was sympathetic and his room was nice and warm.

The stress which Sam's deafness was to cause only gradually came to the surface. In this way Sam and Julia psychosocially constructed 'deafness as a difference' as a 'stress' factor within their relationship. This stress factor appeared in both their private relationship and in their interactions with the outside world. Julia and Sam explored the problem together. Julia began:

> [Sometimes] ... you've misunderstood what I have said, and I get angry because you get angry, and then I make it worse because I say, 'What do you *think* I said? which is awful really ... because it kind of reinforces that he didn't understand in the first place.

Neither Sam nor Julia made any attempt to dodge the difficulties which they experienced. Anyone could get 'the wrong end of the stick' from time to time, but it was more difficult when one partner was profoundly deaf, and the other simultaneously profoundly impatient! Sam replied with understanding:

> Sometimes [people] just don't have the patience ... or communication [skill], ... it's more [about] understanding ... the other person ... When two people live together, they are bound to rub each other up the wrong way now and again.

Sam knew that 'differences' could be managed constructively. Julia occasionally forgot that she must slow down her speech for Sam who was deeply sensitive especially where she was concerned. Julia blamed her unpredictable moods for her occasional incapacity to respond to Sam's 'special needs'. Her insecure background and job often made *her* the demanding one. This was particularly true when there was a crisis. Julia recalled:

> if there's a problem, ... if something has to be arranged or discussed in a hurry, .. it's difficult to translate that quickly to Sam ... I think it is because he is deaf and not because of his personality ...

In such circumstances, Julia experienced Sam's deafness as a 'brick wall' and a stress factor within their relationship. Sam's deafness could also cause stress with strangers in that it provoked rudeness. Sarah recalled how even a so-called friend had made the stupid quip:

> It must be strange for Sam to have sex with you because he can't hear your ecstasy.

Julia forgave people for such intrusiveness, but it also made her feel uncomfortable and sad.

What was distinctive about Sam and Julia's relationship was its complete lack of pretence. Moreover, they were both very open about the negative impact of deafness on their lives, and made no attempt to glamorize or trivialize it. Julia deeply experienced the 'stress' along with Sam although she knew she occasionally provoked it. This meant that Sam was not left to handle it alone unless it was his choice to do so. Sam expressed his appreciation of Julia's enduring support by saying from the heart. 'She gave me back my youth.'

Sam, understandably, felt enormous gratitude towards Julia. In most, although not all situations she was able to prevent the 'stressful' side of 'deafness as a difference' from tainting their enjoyment of life and of each other. A similar sense of gratitude was experienced by Joe in his relationship with Sarah now described.

Fortuitous circumstances: Sarah and Joe

Joe, a designer, divorced after a twenty year marriage and father of two sons, recalled:

> In my first marriage, the woman, although she was encouraging, wasn't understanding enough about the problem of communication ... so much so that [her attitude] was passed on to my sons ...

Joe blamed his first wife for not helping his sons to understand the implications of his deafness for effective communication. Sarah, his new wife, added reflectively:

> I suppose your biggest 'if only' is that there had been someone who was able to explain to your wife what your problem was so that your wife could explain to your boys ...

Sarah thought that sympathetic counselling might have saved Joe's marriage. Because his disability had been largely denied by Joe's first family, it was very important that Sarah and Joe shared a common understanding of it in this second attempt at matrimony. They both found reassurance in Sarah's profession as a lip-reading teacher, seeing it as a guarantee that the meaning of 'deafness as a difference' within their relationship would be psychosocially constructed as a 'communication problem'. While Sarah obviously felt that the extra effort required to communicate with Joe was worthwhile, she did experience real deficits especially the loss of spontaneous chat. Sarah related:

> in the kitchen [I] am sitting at the table ... literally wait[ing] until Joe has finished moving around ... I am not complaining because he is usually ... helping, ... [but] you can't ... say silly things like 'We've run out of milk' when your head's in the fringe ... there's no point.

Sarah pointed to what I have conceptualized as the ETTA factor. This was the Effort, Time, Thought and Attention required by

Sarah so that Joe could lip-read her. The concept of ETTA draws attention to the fact that some hearing people must think carefully about the requirements for lip-reading. This is because what they feel to be their natural and normal way of speaking runs counter to these requirements. Specifically they have to think whether or not at a particular point in time they have the energy to put into the Effort, Time, Thought and Attention needed to engage with a lip-reading hearing impaired person (Schlesinger, 1985). Sarah explained that more time was required when communicating with hearing impaired people because 'you've got to be more graphic ... to use a lot more visual signs'.

Sarah's previous marriage had alerted her that communication as well as love was needed to make a marriage work (Satir, 1972). But Joe's hearing impairment made the situation more complex. She first explained her conception of normality:

> well 'normal' means fast speedy conversation, not thinking about whether it's lip-readable or audible, [or] if the light's on your face, ... [or] you talk like this [putting your hand over your mouth] ... [Normal conversation means] talking while you're eating your cheese sandwich, while you're reading your paper ... that's absolutely normal ...

The ETTA factor is about taking the trouble to accommodate to what does *not* feel normal. It is about having the energy for the Effort, Time, Thought, and Attention required to help a hearing impaired person take their rightful place in both formal and informal conversations. The provision of access to conversations follows the same principle as the provision of a ramp for wheelchair users so that they may enter and leave buildings. This concept will be reintroduced in the next chapter in the context of 'caring'. Sarah also mentioned how inhibiting Joe's deafness could be when they were in bed. She recalled:

> when Joe takes his hearing aids out at night, he's gone ... absolutely gone ... I don't feel alone, but I always think it will become quite a big effort to become intimate and I find that quite difficult because I like to express things ...

Sarah's experience echoed Debbie Kisor's (1990) as they both saw the inability to hear as an obstacle to intimate communication. Their attitudes may be contrasted to that of hearing people who are the sons and daughters of deaf parents (Preston, 1994). Although there is much variation, many of them had learned in their childhoods that darkness and silence did not necessarily preclude communication especially that conveyed through forms of touch.

The psychosocial constructions of 'deafness as a difference' have been discussed for four of the five couples mentioned in this chapter. For the fifth couple, Barbara and Ben, 'deafness as a difference' psychosocially constructed as a 'frustration' was not conceptualized until after their children were born.

The integration of 'deafness as a difference' varied in degree with each marriage and was examined with care, since sometimes what couples said was not what they did (Jones, 1984).

At the next stage, couples continued to work on their mutual psychosocial construction of 'deafness as a difference', but other concerns took priority.

Stage II: Getting serious

Significant others

Stage II began when couples told 'significant others' of their attachment and of the definite possibility of future commitment. The percentage of cohabiting couples in the study appeared to reflect the national norm of just over half of courting couples (Dormor, 1990). Of the five couples discussed in this chapter, three cohabited from three months to one year before they married. One couple married a little more quickly than intended as the wife was pregnant; and the fifth couple, where both partners were training for the ministry, had a traditional wedding ceremony.

Meeting one's future in-laws is a stage that most newly formed couples find daunting, but the risks taken by partners when one is hearing and the other is hearing impaired are greater. This is because couples are drawn from two groups, sociologically speaking, 'outsiders' and 'insiders', and may be perceived as deviant and unacceptable by either group (Higgens, 1980).

Arthur and Gwen were the only couple in the study to explain this developmental stage in detail, as they had married a relatively short period before the time of interviewing. Arthur remembered:

> [Gwen's] parents ... were very encouraging ... [In the past when] I had been taken home to a girl's parents, ... a few of them had not been very welcoming, because I am deaf, and especially with a history of deafness in the family.

Gwen's parents were exceptional as reflected in their attempt to learn BSL. Gwen's mother, Beatrice, recalled her feelings about Arthur and his deafness when they first met:

> [Arthur's] deafness was never an ... obstacle. [He] was welcomed in just as any boyfriend [of Gwen's] would be welcomed in, and we made allowances ...

Beatrice acknowledged a sense of enrichment:

> [Arthur's] coming into our family has opened a completely new world for us and we have learned a great deal from Judy and Paul, his parents.

Beatrice thought their welcoming attitude might be connected to a tradition of 'hospitality' which she and her husband, Andrew, had experienced growing up on the Isle of Lewis. Arthur also introduced Gwen to his parents during this stage, as they lived near her first teaching post, but he gave them less preparation. Gwen recounted:

> [He] introduced me as 'this is Gwen: can she come and live with you in September?' which his mother accepted ... I had his room ... it was useful for me because it improved my Signing.

Arthur's assurance of his parent's cooperation under such circumstances is perhaps indicative of the depth of trust which existed in this Deaf family. What occurred next may be interpreted as Arthur and Gwen's version of a cultural exchange programme with romantic overtones.

At this time in their courtship, Arthur lived in Gwen's house in Reading so that he could finish his college course and Gwen lived in Arthur's home in Southampton so she could begin her teaching job. Although there were practical reasons for this arrangement, it provided Gwen and Arthur with an excellent opportunity to experience the family culture (Reiss, 1981) in which the other partner had grown up. It was also a way of coming to terms with differences in a direct manner right from the beginning. Gwen and Arthur recalled their experiences. Gwen began:

> Your Mom's house is much more structured than mine ... I had to be tidier ... I found from time to time I was called to the door ... [and] I would be the interpreter ... it was difficult for me to work out how much to get involved in that sort of thing ... [As for loss of sound], ... I missed the radio in the mornings dreadfully because we in Reading get up to Radio 4, ... and it really pushes you out the door ... [In the end], I got used to it.

Gwen's brief experience with Arthur's parents reflected descriptions of what it is like growing up as a hearing child with Deaf parents (Preston, 1994). Like them she had to struggle with mixed feelings about silence and the responsibility of interpretation. Arthur gave his account:

> [living with Gwen's parents] affected them more than it affected me ... [as I had already become] familiar [with hearing people] ... the only adjustment I had to make was to adapt to ... household rules ... since two households are never alike.

In-laws were reported as being important at this stage by two other couples. Ben did not refer to Barbara's severe deafness when he first introduced her to his parents as he wished them to meet Barbara, 'the person' not Barbara the 'deaf girl'. While Ben's attitude was commendable up to a point, Barbara had been deaf a long time. There was the question as to why it had to be 'either/or' rather than both Barbara, the person *and* Barbara, the deaf girl. The uncon-scious message conveyed was that Barbara the deaf girl was someone repulsive who belonged outside family boundaries. Full integration could not take place because apparently neither Barbara, Ben, or his parents could cope with the mixed feelings caused by acknowledging that Barbara was both normal and different, hearing and deaf.

Management of interpersonal power

The couple's feelings about the developing power balance was also investigated. Much is written in the sociological literature about power in interpersonal relationships (Bernard, 1982; Eichler, 1981). Interpersonal power here refers to the ability to achieve a desired end through influence. In other words, power enters a relationship when people (i.e. powerholders) have the ability to achieve ends by influencing others. The literature suggests a number of interper-sonal power models. French and Raven (1962) list six different types of power bases which people use in their interpersonal relations: reward, coercive, referent, legitimate, expert and informational. Traditionally men are viewed as using a greater number of power bases than women, but this is changing. For example, Scanzoni and Scanzoni (1981) identify two marriage models: (a) the corporation type of marriage where the husband acts the role of chief executive with the wife as junior partner: (b) the egalitarian marriage where there is relative equality between the spouses rights and privileges. They both have full-time careers and share in all decisions.

Power problems at this stage connected with 'deafness as a difference' must seem manageable or the relationship will flounder. Arthur and Gwen reflected on this point. Arthur said:

> one important characteristic [of our relationship] is that it's a partnership of equals, rather than a partnership where one partner dominates the other ... we have our particular strengths and weaknesses. And if I have a weakness, [Gwen] has a strength which compensates, and vice versa ...

Undoubtedly, Arthur and Gwen shared a vision of a relationship which could be interdependent (Weingarten, 1978) rather than the carer/cared for, dependent/independent model (Parker, 1993; Oliver, 1990). Arthur also took care to be discriminating and by the use of understatement, he inferred that hearing people were not superior just because they were hearing, as his Deaf parents supposed. Gwen continued the theme confirming the concept of need-complementarity (Rosow, 1957):

> We have had different experiences, but we can put those together. I had been through college, and Arthur had not ... so that made me all the more determined to help him ...

However, Arthur's job preferences were changing. He recalled:

> I had this irrational fear of telling ... [Gwen] that I now wanted to be an accountant and not a social worker. [Perhaps] ... if I had told her, our relationship ... would suffer ... or she might call off the wedding ... so I kept quiet about it ...

The fact that Arthur should have doubted the strength of Gwen's commitment to him was understandable given the long history of hearing people's neglect of Deaf people's welfare (Lane, 1984: Wright, 1990). Gwen expressed her exasperation at Arthur's inability to trust her:

> I ... don't mind what he does. I will support him in anything as long as I know in which direction we are going, ... it was [his] not telling me that I didn't like ...

Gwen had the potential to be a powerful healer as she not only symbolized 'woman as helpmate', she also brought the hope of equality with hearing people. There were moments, however, when Gwen increased Arthur's anxiety such as when she refused to accept his proposal of marriage until he had a job, and when she was half an hour late for their wedding.

Henry had similar thoughts about his relationship with Kay. He recalled:

> being a deaf person [with a hearing] partner ... at the beginning of the marriage, I used to feel quite insecure when we got in to an area of tension. I always felt because she was 'hearing', she had the upper hand; but because of the way Kay is as a person, she's allowed me to go through the experience and mature ...

Henry was very appreciative of the support which Kay gave him. However, the real issue between the couples generally was not of 'equality' in the abstract, but how the hearing spouses with their command of English actually managed their linguistic power with their hearing impaired partners (Barbara, 1989).

An exchange between Arthur and Gwen typified what could occur. They were discussing what kind of education their unborn child ought to have. Eventually Arthur became fed up with Gwen's dogmatic tone and said:

> You never ... gave me a chance [to explain myself properly] ... I felt [you were] almost accusing ... me [of not caring] ... about [our] children's emotional development, or their ability to think.

While Arthur was careful to be respectful of Gwen and her expert professional teacher power base, he felt hurt by her apparent disregard for his opinion in his roles as her husband and the future father of their children (Doyle and Paludi, 1991). Gwen clarified her attitude:

> I'm not saying you don't care, but that I worry that the type of school you want, won't care ... You ... are ready to find out about these schools, I've already formed my opinion.

Although Arthur could fight back, it was not without a certain amount of anguish. While Gwen was inflexible here, Arthur could be equally so, especially on the topic of sign language and the past treatment of Deaf people.

Hearing partners in this book appeared gradually to learn to restrain their linguistic power for they valued an egalitarian relationship with their hearing impaired partners. Surprisingly, this power was not necessarily the prerogative of the hearing partner. For example, Robert, deafened as he approached retirement from Menière's Disease, was more articulate than his hearing wife, Mary. Rachel, who suffered from otosclerosis, spoke more forcefully than her hearing husband, Richard.

When some of these issues had begun to be addressed, the couples gradually moved to Stage III where they become more self-consciously 'a couple'.

Stage III: Making it work

While the themes of Stage I and II continue, there are new issues as the couples' relationships move into the stage of commitment. The couples begin to settle down and to become more aware of what it uniquely means to be 'a couple', and to respect that meaning. They begin to explore the various social structures surrounding them which can help take the stressful edge off a marriage relationship where 'deafness as a difference' is being integrated. Routines are established, social networks evaluated and developed, and new leisure/work patterns explored. The couples learn that stress and crises will continue, as in all marriages, and that they are manageable as patterns of support begin to emerge and warning signs seen.

Issues faced by the emerging couple

Experiencing stress

As we have seen, the meaning of Sam's profound deafness was psychosocially constructed as 'stressful'. It provoked rudeness in others and enormous frustration in Julia especially in times of crisis. An area of 'stress' for Sarah and Joe was 'disclosure' when they were out shopping as they had very different attitudes about it. Joe recalled:

> I wanted to get a pair of ... binoculars ... We found a nice shop ... and I ... [went] in and ... [started] talking to the young [sales] man ... But I ... [didn't] tell him I'm hard of hearing ...

As a traditionally socialized male, Joe was reluctant to disclose as he wished to avoid the condescending attitudes his past disclosures had provoked. Sarah found his behaviour frustrating as she explained:

> But it's interesting as an observer how ... relieved people are when they know someone [is] hard of hearing, ... rather than having to spend ... [time] trying to explain something and thinking, [when the communication breaks down that] it's them[selves], or thinking they're facing a stupid man ...

Sarah's 'common sense' view was also understandable. She confided:

> Now ... when ... [Joe] is having an interaction in a shop, I move away, ... [otherwise] they always end up talking to me ...

Because of their differing attitudes, Sarah had learned that it was best to withdraw completely from the situation. Gwen talked about the stress she experienced during her first year of marriage to Arthur:

> The doctor said, 'Oh you have just got married, go get on with it' sort of thing ... And then it passed over ... I had just finished my first year of teaching ... so it was all a bit much in one go.

Eventually Gwen and Arthur discovered that an established routine helped cut down their anxiety. Feelings of stress were also attached to interpreting tasks. Here Gwen talked about making telephone calls for Arthur:

> I get exasperated in having to make phone calls for him. I hate it ... I don't know why.

Arthur agreed:

> This [situation] upsets me [too], because if my hearing was OK, I'd be doing the phoning, and it upsets me that other people seem reluctant to phone [on my behalf].

This switch in natural talent made them both feel extremely uncomfortable within their relationship resulting in further stressful feelings.

Arthur and Gwen had already begun to work out a more appropriate solution in the context of ordering meals when eating out. Gwen explained:

> [Arthur] used to rely on me ... when we went to a restaurant. I was giving the order ... and people would look at him as if he were peculiar or something ... there's nothing wrong with his speech ... I make him do it now and it's fine ... but you didn't like it, did you?

Arthur replied:

> I hated it ... I felt silly, self conscious, ... but it's not so bad now.

Arthur was prepared to overcome his anxiety to please Gwen. She in turn was sensitive to Arthur's 'situational dependence', sensing when to act, and when to encourage him to risk possible embarrassment.

A mutual vision of interpendence and commitment

Mansfield and Collard (1991) maintain that despite present diversity in contemporary social life, there are two basic issues at the heart of becoming and remaining a couple: commitment and interdependence. Commitment may be seen as a belief that stabilizes the behaviour of couples in that they have faith in their long-term relationship. Other scholars are more blunt and see commitment as perseverance stemming from a balance between a 'have to' (cost) and 'want to' (reward) (Scanzoni *et al.*, 1989).

The concept of interdependence as a measure of a marital relationship is relatively new. Cohen (1974) writes that it is rather a bargain ... between two adequate, self-sufficient, successfully dependent adults, namely that the giving goes both ways. In terms of coping with dependency needs, the equilibrium (achieved) must be flexible enough to allow for shifts in situations of stress.

If two people are to be defined as ' a couple', there needs to be a level of interdependence in at least some of the following dimensions: sexual, economic, emotional, practical and social. Sarah and Joe had a very clear conception of what they could give and take from a marriage relationship. Sarah explained:

> when I got married [to Joe], I said I'm not going to do any more housework, and no more Sunday lunches ... a waste of time. Someone else can do it who likes to see things clean ...

This didn't worry Joe as he was delighted to have found a partner who understood his 'special needs', who was so hospitable and caring and who had experienced loss herself without being devastated by it. He said:

> I went through a rotten experience being deaf, Sarah also went through a rotten experience and we've met and disproved how difficult it is for a deaf person to get on with a hearing person ...

Joe and Sarah built a relationship around physical attraction, common interests, mutual experiences of 'loss' and continuing support. This formed the basis of the commitment and interdependence that satisfied them. The nature of commitment emerged with another couple, Julia and Sam, as they explored the possibility of Sam having a cochlear implant operation. Julia explained:

> but if Sam had [the operation], and that's what he wanted, ... I would be very pleased for him ... Sam supports me and I support him so I would support whatever he wanted to do ... unless he wanted to run off with somebody else ...

Julia's slightly frivolous remark did not belie her devotion. Arthur also struggled to articulate his feelings about his and Gwen's relationship:

> in 18 months the equality of the bond [between us] has changed ... I think we are much more dependent on each other. I'd have said we don't need anybody else, ... yes [we've become] a couple instead of two people ... we have become an entity ...

Gwen had a more earthy perspective for she replied:

> Well we argue less, but again that's ... because we are coping better with all the stress ... when we first got married ... we just argued all the time ...

Arthur and Gwen, as they became more committed and involved with each other, discovered that some old ties had loosened. They went on to consider the specific nature of their relationships with closer relations and friends.

Initial social network formation

As two individuals become a couple, they begin to make sense of the social world around them (Finch, 1989). Families of origin appeared to play an important role in initial social network formation. Sarah and Joe were proud of the links which had been maintained with

Sarah's family. Barbara and Ben mentioned that they had 'invested' a lot in their families of origin.

Julia and Sam had mixed feelings about their families, but were glad they were there. Henry and Kay had found strength in the feeling that they were both from the same type of middle-class background. Besides family, Gwen was aware that her relationship with her best friend, Charity, had taken on a new dimension after she had decided to marry Arthur. She recalled:

> My best friend ... [of] ten years, ... Charity, ... she is single ... She thinks [Arthur's] wonderful, but if [we get together], it's Charity and I, [who] go off together ... we leave [Arthur behind], ... because ... he'd be bored to death. She and I are like another couple ... a different sort of couple.

Gwen was able to retreat into a more familiar same sex hearing relationship with a single friend. Having gained strength, she was able to cope with the demands of her marriage. Arthur, on the other hand, did not require such a relationship which he interpreted as a gender difference between them (Allan, 1989).

Making new friends

Couples who have normalized 'deafness as a difference' in their relationships are likely to puzzle people generally. Their social world is complex with potential for both enrichment and rejection.

Prelingually deaf Barbara, illustrated this point with her realistic assessment of the difficulties. She felt that busy hearing people were often wary of her as they did not know what burdens friendship with her might bring. Because of this, she often took social initiatives as she believed that this strategy helped to counteract the possibility that she would be seen as a 'wounded bird'. Although her hearing husband, Ben, was aware of Barbara's struggle, his role was usually to support from the sidelines.

In fact, the women in this study, whether deaf or hearing, appeared to feel responsible for initiating new friendships. Gwen reflected:

> I don't ... find it easy to make [new] friends ... I'm lucky that I've ... acquired enough over the years ... twice we went to the pub with all these young teachers, and they just ignored ... [Arthur]. Well I won't put up with that ... he comes first, ... and if they don't want to know him then I don't want to know them.

Arthur's immediate come back was:

> If people start to be funny about Gwen, then I would shut them out ... the only
> relationship that matters is ours.

Gwen and Arthur were concerned about the possibility of encountering 'stigma' from members of their own cultural/work group
directed towards their partner (Higgens, 1980). They found it less
stressful to make acquaintances and friends in the local branch of an
organization called 'The Breakthrough Trust'. It encouraged hearing and Deaf people to meet and contained a number of couples like
themselves. Gwen recalled making one new friend using the time-
honoured method of 'secret sharing' (Tannen, 1991):

> The closest friend I've made is a colleague at work, ... she is old enough to be
> my mother ... I've told her about the baby, I haven't told anybody else ... she's
> very good to me ...

As a bicultural couple, Gwen and Arthur began to discover where
they were and were not welcome. Their attitudes appeared the
reverse of what might be expected. Although Arthur was Deaf, it was
Gwen who appeared to have the greater fear of rejection and the
lower self-esteem. She acknowledged how her advocacy role with
Deaf people, specifically with Arthur and his family, helped her to
overcome her fears:

> Oh yes, I could do anything if it's for them ... [Arthur] or his Mum ... But if it's
> for myself, I won't do it [like] asking for things in shops ... [I'd rather] go out
> empty-handed. [Their need] gives me something to hide behind.

Gwen had stumbled on the circular nature of help in that there was
an interdependence not just between herself and Arthur and his
family, but between Deaf and hearing people more generally
(Higgens, 1980; Preston, 1994). Social networks will be discussed in
greater detail in Chapters 8 and 9.

Summary

Here the five partners who committed themselves to each other
when one partner was already severely/profoundly hearing
impaired are discussed. There is the suggestion that the deafness was

unconsciously if not consciously part of the attraction. It was found that these relationships developed over three stages.

Stage I (Meeting and Liking) began when the hearing partners reassured their hearing impaired partners that their 'special needs' were manageable. Partners also had to construct mutually and psychosocially the meaning of 'deafness as a difference'. In other words, an anthropological/cultural perspective rather than a medical model was used. This highly personal joint perception was then integrated into their growing relationship. For example, the five couples psychosocially constructed deafness to have five different meanings: 'an insignificant factor', 'respectable and OK', 'a communication problem', 'a stress factor' and 'a frustration'. These constructions appeared to occur unconsciously because of the emotional 'fit' between the partners, but were consciously acknowledged in the couples' professed ability to talk easily and openly with each other. At this stage, some hearing partners became aware of the ETTA factor (Effort, Thought, Time and Attention), or the requirements needed for their hearing impaired partner to lip read. Other partners, for example Ben, had sufficiently integrated these requirements so they were unconscious.

In Stage II (Getting Serious) the partners took their infant relationship to 'significant others'. The expectation was that family members might be threatened. This was found to be the case with some families, but not with others. During that time, couples also evaluated the interpersonal power balance in their relationship. The majority of couples described themselves implicitly if not explicitly as being egalitarian, committed and interdependent. The issue of 'dependence' was found to be a situational phenomenon within a continuing reciprocal relationship.

Stage III (Making It Work) began as couples became more earnest in their intentions, often seeking a formal as well as informal expression of their commitment. Various social structures developed around them which helped to balance the formidable side of 'deafness as a difference' within their relationship. As the couples felt more secure and less tense with their shared perception of 'deafness as a deafness', they were able to bring some order into their family responsibilities and friendship. These couples needed very specific listening and communicating skills because of the enormous scope for misunderstanding. The very nature of 'deafness as a difference' in their marriages meant that the people in this book came into contact sooner than other couples with areas of conflict. In most cases, there was sufficient love, wisdom and communication skill to manage them.

Since similar perspectives and experiences could not be assumed, a process of like-mindedness had to be nurtured. The problems of such a marriage were by nature the same as those of an ordinary marriage, but they were experienced earlier, had greater intensity and had more significant consequences. The distinctiveness necessary at the heart of such a relationship was what made it special. In making allowances at the very beginning of the relationship for ways the other person was different, pleasure for both partners was created as they became aware of the variety in their relationship. It enabled a husband or wife to say everyday, 'He/she never ceases to surprise me' (Barbara, 1989: 211).

We now consider the impact of hearing impairment on the continuing relationships. Some of the couples in this chapter will be revisited.

CHAPTER 5

Continuing couple relationships

Introduction

The five couples just discussed will now be revisited in the light of their continuing relationship along with six new couples whose hearing impairment did not occur until their marriages were well established. Consequently none of the partners in this latter group had entered their marriage expecting to need or to provide any extra care as a result of a disability, such as deafness. We will now explore how the sudden traumatic 'loss' of hearing in one partner within a continuing committed relationship affected that relationship.

The fact that the disability requiring adjustment did not occur until the marriage was well established has parallels with the experiences of couples discussed by Parker (1993). There are also differences, however, in that the behaviour of the six couples in this chapter fits the anthropological/cultural model in much the same way as emerged in Chapter 4, rather than a medical model. This is because the disabled partner did not require traditional forms of 'tending care' (Bulmer, 1987) as emerged in Parker's study. For these mutual perceptions to develop, a new 'contract' had to be implicitly negotiated by the couples which incorporated the realities of the degree, type and nature of hearing impairment along with methods for coping with it.

In order to understand how the couples negotiated or renegotiated their contracts, the concept of 'care' needs to be assessed along with the sociological context from which it develops. 'Care' on an intuitive level is described as the provision of help, support, and protection for vulnerable and dependent members of society. A strong distinction is made between 'care' as concern about people generally and the actual looking after or the 'tending' of more or less dependent people.

Bulmer (1987) suggests that 'care' may be seen on a spectrum of three types, with each type being further removed from the recipient of the care. Firstly, there is the physical 'tending care' just described. Secondly, there is material and psychological support which does not involve physical contact, such as the telephone support given from kin and friends to an elderly person. Lastly, there is a more generalized concern about the welfare of others which may or may not lead to the other two types of help.

There are, of course, connections between the help which hearing impaired people receive from their partner and traditional concepts of 'care' to be interpreted as 'the roles' adopted by the hearing partner on behalf of the hearing impaired partner as the situation required. However, there are a number of difficulties in making this connection. Firstly, the help provided by the able-bodied partner, the hearing spouse for the hearing impaired spouse, rarely caused the distress (Ungerson, 1987) mentioned in the Parker study; although on occasion in certain specific situations, the findings suggest that stress, frustration and resentment occurred. In acknowledging this, it is understood that stress, frustration and resentment occur in every close relationship as they are natural responses in coming to grips with human differences. Many would argue that the institution of marriage itself brings about negative feelings to an extreme degree as partially evidenced by the high divorce rate (Clark and Haldane, 1990). Secondly, 'care' was never provided on an all consuming daily basis, but only occasionally when needed for specific situations. Thirdly, the hearing impaired member of every couple was employed in a paid or volunteer capacity, and able to function in the public sphere completely independently of their partner. In contrast to other studies (Preston, 1994), which imply that such relationships cannot be reciprocal (Gouldner, 1960), in the long term, a loving rapport on both sides is the most significant and striking feature of most of the study couples. Initially, however, it is not always evident how the eight people with the more severe/profound losses in the study returned the social access support that was so obviously and generously given.

The majority of couples studied presented aspects of the 'ideal' companionate marriage described by Berger and Kellner (1964) in that partners were close enough to perceive and construct reality together (Foster, 1989). A similar idea has been applied to the way in which families construct the reality around them (Reiss, 1981).

But unlike the Berger and Kellner model, couples described here also presented more realistic aspects of their relationship (Morgan, 1981) resulting from a deep understanding of the demands and constraints of society, two careers, children, and the disability itself. Therefore, the type of marriage which emerged contained a balance of realistic and idealistic aspects reflecting some understanding of both the institutional and relational components of marriage similar to the couples interviewed by Mansfield and Collard (1988).

Finally, because marriage is a relational system, this study adopts the 'Epigenetic Principle' (Wynne, 1988) introduced in Chapter 3 for examining the ways in which hearing loss affects couples. According to this developmental principle, there are five relational processes. In this chapter, there will be a detailed analysis of the first relational process: attachment/caregiving. Chapter 6 develops the analysis continuing the use of the Epigenetic Principle. Here the focus will be on the advanced processes: 'communication', 'problem-solving', and 'mutuality'. Intimacy, the most developed relational problem, is discussed in Chapter 3.

First relational process: attachment and caregiving

An understanding of attachment/caregiving processes is largely drawn from John Bowlby's theory of 'attachment and loss'. The fact that attachment behaviour is less obvious when the affectional bonds are felt to be secure, does not mean that the underlying affectional bonds are less. Ainsworth comments that 'in a good marriage each partner on occasion plays the role of the stronger and wiser figure for the other, so that each derives security and comfort from the other, as well as wishing to be with the other and protesting against actual or threatened separation' (1982: 26).

It might, therefore, be expected that the married hearing impaired people in the study would be strongly attached to their hearing partners. It might also be assumed that the attachment would be stronger when the hearing loss was greater. Some people's remarks suggested this. Henry, a severely hearing impaired theological student acknowledged:

> Kay is ... a very strong person and has a deep Christian commitment [and] faith ... a very moral person ... she gives me a tremendous amount of strength and security to enable me to come up ...

Although Kay was not as generous with her praise, she was especially thankful for Henry's presence during specific moments such as when she gave birth to their second child:

> Yes, I'm afraid I was very much physically hanging on to Henry as keeping me in reality [during labour]; and as he was there, everything would be all right eventually.

Kay lacked appreciation of how her vulnerability in this instance nourished the reciprocity in her relationship with Henry. Reciprocity was displayed more openly by Joe and Sarah. Joe recalled:

> Sarah has done a tremendous amount for me, as she is doing for a lot of people ... [and she] brought new life into mine.

Sarah tempered her enthusiasm with realism:

> the last ten years ... have been the happiest in my life ... I don't say that I don't get fed up 'coz Joe knows I do, ... [but] now we overcome it by talking about it ... and we never have nasty in-depth rows.

As emerged in Chapter 4, Sarah was more than happy to cope with what they had mutually perceived as their 'communication problem' or the meaning of Joe's deafness, if in exchange, Joe was prepared to talk things through in contrast to the rowing pattern she had encountered in past failed relationships.

Deafened Sam and his hearing partner, Julia, were the first to admit that they did have rows. However, they appeared to resemble lover's tiffs in that it was safe to row without causing permanent damage. She explained her enormous regard for Sam:

> [Sam] ... is the victim of ... [the GP who prescribed the drug that deafened him], who made a gross error ... it's only Sam's personality and his strength of character which has helped him keep on an even keel, .. through going deaf and living with it.

Julia was openly admiring of Sam's stoic tenacity and refusal to become embittered when he became the victim of a doctor's ignorance. Sam, in turn, talked about his enjoyment of Julia's company:

> When we lived in Norfolk, we were together the whole day and the whole evening ... we got on all right ... What I would like ... [is to own] a small ... farm ... if we both worked on that, we would see each other all day, but we wouldn't be in each other's pockets.

The above quotations reveal the reciprocity of attachment found generally within the relationships of the couples in this study. Two deafened spouses stood out in that their praise of their hearing spouses was more restrained. Joy remarked offhandedly:

> Well, of course I've had my husband to help me through; and we've carried on more or less like we've always done.

Joy's remarks suggested that her enforced social dependency (Scott, 1969) on Mike had caused her to value him less, a phenomenon noted by Hetu, Jones and Getty (1993). Anthony, from Nigeria, talked in a teasing tone about his hearing wife, Clare:

> She is a good girl ... not as good as before ... she's changed ... she's no more good ... I'm joking ... there are many qualities ... the way she talks, the way she takes life, ... the company of goodness ...

The joking ambivalent tone of Anthony's initial remarks can be better understood by a closer look at his and Clare's cultural context. Anthony was likely to be reflecting the strong 'macho' element in Nigerian, specifically Ibo culture. His words also revealed his frustration and displeasure at his dependence on Clare for 'interpretation' in social situations, which he had previously easily controlled with his enormous charm and warmth. Such feelings are not restricted to deafened African men since they are well documented as experienced in the UK (Kyle, Jones and Wood, 1985).

Clare didn't take offence at Anthony's initial disparaging tone because she knew his life was difficult and that he had compensating qualities for his occasional irritability, especially his genuinely responsible and caring attitude towards his family. Unlike some wives (Lamb, Pleck and Levine, 1987), Clare was happily aware of her good fortune in being married to such a man.

Anthony, himself, believed that his deafness had made him more responsible and more serious. Nevertheless, his seriousness was tempered with humour. Clare recalled:

> Yes, Anthony has a good sense of humour ... a crazy sense of humour ... it makes [our relationship fun]. [It helps to] laugh it off ...

The focus now moves to the more general area of domestic sociability.

Domestic sociability

Domestic sociability is defined here as the spontaneous expressive remarks, sometimes humorous, to do with the practical, social and current events of the day. This type of exchange is not especially profound, but is often intrinsically gratifying in that it conveys belonging (Blau, 1967), and is seen as a cohesive force in relationships especially among women (Tannen, 1991; Schloch, 1988). These exchanges could be on the level where most marital conversation takes place; or could be the first rung of a deeper relational process, for example, communication or a type of intimacy.

From earlier discussions, Sarah and Joe will be remembered for perceiving Joe's severe deafness as a 'communication problem'. Throughout the interviews, Sarah frequently recalled her feelings of 'loss' in conversing spontaneously with Joe. She pointed out that Joe's deafness, and a number of his more formidable mannerisms, inhibited her desire to launch both serious discussions as well as more inconsequential ones. She recalled:

> Well, it stops you talking ... [and] making remarks about what's in the papers and [you] think, 'Oh, I cannot be bothered' ... but I haven't got the energy sometimes ...

While Joe also shared a sense of 'loss', it seemed to be a more general feeling about life. He explained:

> I quite like to forget ... that I can't live a [completely] normal life ... although I keep on saying, Let's keep it 'normal' ... it's not [always] possible.

While Sarah sometimes felt socially deprived, these feelings lessened with time as confirmed by Parker (1993). The feelings of sadness lessened as the ETTA (Effort, Thought, Time and Attention) factor required for effective communication with Joe was integrated.

Other hearing spouses mentioned similar feelings with regard to loss of spontaneity. Mary (68) and Robert (70) deafened from Menières, were both retired school teachers. Mary remarked:

> Sometimes [while watching television], I miss sharing things ... Although ... [we're] watching it together, ... you can't have television and talking.

Mike agreed, but referred specifically to the use of subtitles. He said:

> While the subtitling is on, ... I can't talk to [Joy] ... because if she looks at me [so she can lip-read], she's missed what's on the television. So you tend to lose out on spontaneity ... I can't have a joke or anything like that while a programme's on ...

For Julia, partner of deafened Sam, there was also a feeling of 'loss' even though she had never actually known Sam when he was hearing. She felt that many of her witty, sarcastic and subtle comments fell flat or were missed. This did not mean they did not appreciate humour together, but it was more visual than oral.

A common pattern emerged in reviewing the couples discussed here. Hearing women married to deaf or deafened men gave something extra, ETTA, to the relationship because they felt something 'special' was given in return. As career women, they particularly appreciated the support and encouragement provided by responsible and caring husbands. Mike and Joy revealed a different pattern which will be discussed in the next section.

The underlying theme of attachment and caregiving will continue as the focus shifts to the specific roles of the hearing partner.

Additional caring roles of the hearing partner

Roles which the hearing partners on occasion carried for their hearing impaired partners were buffer, monitor, interpreter, mediator, prompter, advocate and editor. Their implementation was seen to create a more expressive intensity between the partners than might normally be expected within traditional reserved English middle-class couples. Frustration was sometimes experienced when the hearing impaired partner felt that their hearing partner was not conducting these roles exactly right. There could also be a certain 'social dependency' (Scott, 1969) in such relationships at times. This occasionally resulted in resentment on the part of the hearing impaired spouse and stress on the part of the hearing spouse.

In focusing on these roles, it needs to be restated that the relationship was reciprocal overall. As may be detected in the comments of most partners throughout the book, there was much deep mutual admiration and respect between them. This meant that these roles were taken on within the context of a mutually interdependent and committed relationship. The additional roles may also be seen to reflect appropriate degrees of 'adaptability' found in well optimally functioning family systems (Olson *et al.*, 1983).

The discussion on roles begins with Joy, aged 60, who at the age of 35 was suddenly deafened by Meningitis. She said:

> [Mike] thinks he [understands and] I think he tries to; but, ... sometimes he doesn't seem to realize [how left out I feel], ... [especially] when we are with other people.

Despite Mike fitting the criteria for a 'high marital adjustment husband' (Noller, 1984), interpreting on behalf of Joy was full of pitfalls as she described:

> Sometimes he will realize that I'm not 'in' ... the conversation ... and he will bring me in. But of course, I suppose ... he gets interested in the conversation and will forget about me.

Women may make better interpreters than men. The 'forgetting' attitude mentioned here may go hand in hand with the general flavour of male sociability and bonhomie (Allan, 1989; Orlans, 1985). On the other hand, there are very real complexities as Joy illustrated:

> It is difficult when there are several people ... to bring you into the conversation ... [Mike] will say 'We are talking about something ... ' and I will say 'Oh yes,' and make a remark. And then, of course, a hearing person will pick that up [and I won't be able to hear as the subject changes]. If there are only three, it's not too bad. But more than that ... [is very frustrating].

Mike tried his best in this difficult situation (Cowrie and Douglas-Cowrie, 1987). However, like BSL interpreters, it was likely that he and other spouses of severe/profound hearing impaired people would suffer from 'role strain' on occasion.

Hearing Clare, who had previously interpreted for her Nigerian grandmother, found it much more demanding to interpret for her husband, Anthony. She explained:

> It is ... [a hard] job being an interpreter ... I'm not a very patient person ... so there is a lot of strain ... especially when there's a lively discussion going on, ... it's difficult ... to take part and try to make [Anthony] follow what is being said; ... by the time you've tried telling him what they have said, they've moved on ... I feel guilty when I see him looking lost, and he asks what's going on.

Pauline Ashley made a similar observation about her efforts in helping her husband Jack, the former Labour Member of Parliament, now in the House of Lords. She recalled:

> On social occasions I may be acting as both a participant and an interpreter. It is only too easy to fulfil just one of the roles. I am rather a single-minded person, and, if I get absorbed in conversation, tend to become oblivious of what is going on around me. Fortunately, I have learned to participate in one conversation while simultaneously being aware of another. In this way I can help Jack quickly should it be necessary. (Ashley, 1985: 80)

Although Pauline Ashley implied the possibility of mastering the art of effective social interpreting in time, it seemed doubtful that the stressful element ever really disappears. Sainsbury (1993) suggests some specific reasons for this within a marital as opposed to a professional context; for example, hearing spouses cannot walk away from the problem, they are involved emotionally, they have no official training, they are likely to reproach themselves and be reproached by their spouses for not interpreting quickly or precisely enough, and they don't get paid for it.

Interpretation is seen to be easier if it is shared by other guests in a social situation. For example, Mike mentioned how it worked with friends:

> The husband, because he has a beard, can't talk to Joy directly, ... so it will either be myself that interprets or this other person's wife, Joy's friend ... so there is always some explanation from one or the other of us.

Argyle *et al.*(1968) suggest that women generally are particularly sensitive to nonverbal cues. However, there were occasions when a social evening meant Sarah had additional, sometimes incongruent roles to play. She recalled a particularly embarrassing accident:

> On Saturday evening we had friends here for dinner; and I was bringing through the trolley (from the kitchen). And ... [Joe] asked me a question, ... and ... because I automatically have to turn around to answer [him], the trolley hit the side of the door because I wasn't watching where I was going, ... and unfortunately the cream fell off the trolley ... It ... [wasn't] possible [to be in both roles at once]. I ... couldn't say, 'Wait a minute' or not answer because we had friends here [and that would be rude].

In this instance, Sarah's 'role strain' resulted from the conflict between being a 'hostess' and a 'caring wife' (Jones, Kyle and Wood, 1987).

Along with interpreting, two wives of hearing impaired men also edited their own speech or other people's on behalf of their husbands. However, the reasons for doing this varied. Julia explained her view:

> But there is no way ... [I] ... have the energy sometimes to ... 'precis', ... so that the conversation is ... short, ... meaningful, and to the point. I mean you can't talk about what we call 'the price of tomatoes' forever ... so you need a lot of mental energy.

Joe responded:

> I have no patience with people [who talk about] 'the price of tomatoes'. Please get to the point. Oh no, [I'm not a chatterer] ... A to B finished.

Patience was an issue for both Joe and Sarah, but in opposite activities. While Joe might have chatted more to please Sarah, like many men, he felt more comfortable in conversations which 'reported' rather than feminine 'rapport' talk.

He added:

> [I do communicate socially] but I find, I suppose because I am deaf, I don't like [conversations to be] so long ... that one has to think, 'Now what exactly is that person saying?

Although Joe connected his preferred conversational style with his deafness, it may be a collection of social factors, for example, gender, personality, class and intelligence. Julia also edited for her partner,

Sam, but more in social gatherings than in dyadic conversations. She recalled:

> I ... edit ... for speed [when interpreting] ... so ... complicated sentences ... are ... simplified which can mean that ... [Sam] may lose some of the meaning. Also I may 'interpret' for other people ... sometimes I say things that they have not said to try to get the meaning [across] more quickly ...

Despite Julia's inaccuracies, Sam managed to enter the spirit of these exchanges, doing his best with his own lip-reading skills. Robert (70) deafened by Menières, had a similar strategy when attending the biannual international meeting in France of people with his surname. Mary described what occurred:

> [Robert] starts conversations ... so I come in ... as interpreter, ... [but] Robert's French is ... much better than mine ... [so] we try to work as a team ... I try and understand somebody ... then I tell him, and then he will ... reply, or he will say the first thing and I will hear the answer, and then tell him ... it's sort of [a] three way [process].

Interpreting, editing and prompting are tasks which are often linked with the telephone, an instrument which lip-reading skills cannot currently master. Julia was happy to do Sam's phone work as she was a declared 'phone addict'. She sometimes prompted Sam to speak:

> This is your Mum ... say 'hello' ... and he says 'Hello'.

Sarah regretted doing telephone tasks which she knew Sam preferred, for example, ringing up garages when they wanted a car. Gwen explained how she attempted to approach telephone interpreting from a practical perspective.

> If we were both deaf, ... [Arthur] would find another hearing person to do [the telephoning] ... it's like marrying someone who is good with cars, you never have to worry about the garage bills ...

Other issues connected with the use of the telephone were 'social decision making' and 'privacy'. An example of the latter was when Mike became 'carried away' in accepting or initiating social invitations on the phone. Deafened Joy sometimes resented being told after a conversation was completed that 'so and so' was coming over or the reverse. Joy also felt a sense of loss when Mike answered the phone to her personal friends. She explained:

> my friends call and of course Mike has to answer ... it's not like having a [proper] telephone conversation ... you can't have any secrets ... yes, I do miss the telephone ... it's just [that] other people don't like writing ... I don't belong to the RNID telephone exchange. It's very useful if you've got a business ... but for ordinary chat, it hardly seems worth it ... no privacy.

Mike, like Julia, obviously enjoyed using the telephone so he was happy with his interpreter role. Joy, however, regretted her inability to use the phone as it represented a double loss: an inability to monitor their social life and to retain autonomy over intimate friendships (Doyle and Gough, 1986).

Clare related difficulties about the 'timing' and 'style' of phone calls for Anthony. She complained:

> [Anthony] asks me to phone a friend, ... and all he wants me to do is deliver the message, ... and drop the phone ... I've got to say 'Hello, How do you do? ... How are you getting on? ...

Because Anthony was a recently deafened extrovert man, his inability to make his own phone calls was particularly frustrating. His frustration was compounded by Clare's refusal to make business-like phone calls. Clare continued:

> [Also when] he wants me to make a phone call, it [must be] immediately ... He wants me to drop everything.

This complaint was echoed by Gwen and suggested that for an extrovert male, delayed phone calls were difficult regardless of how long they have been deaf. Thus the complex nature of telephone interpreting stood out as causing more stress and conflict than any other role accepted by the hearing spouse. In this specific situation, it was Anthony who had to adjust, but not without a tinge of resentment. He said:

> if I have to get someone to ... make a telephone call, the people ... [I] work with in my course, they do it better and with more willingess than [my wife, Clare] ...

Anthony, however, was adamant that he and Clare never stored up resentment about their differing attitudes. When discussing their marriage more generally, he talked about how they had learned to negotiate. He said:

> Myself and my wife ... we are both individuals who don't keep [resentments] in the mind for long ... I will only say that ... life continues again ... we go to bed friendly ...

Anthony and Clare, in fact, were involved in a massive emotional and cultural adjustment, a result not only of Anthony's sudden deafness, but also of the losses involved with their migration to England. Both losses imposed at least a temporary discrepancy between inner and outer worlds, which had to be realigned if they were to adapt and survive with any degree of physical and mental health (Huntington, 1984; Freid, 1962).

Mike and Joy, in contrast, were from the same London suburb, but they shared with Anthony and Clare a similar orientation about marriage. Mike remembered:

> We've always done things together ... we've each got money ... it doesn't matter who spends it ... it's ours not mine [nor] Joy's ... so whatever we've got belongs to both of us.

If Mike and Joy shared the prizes of life, they also shared the burdens. Unsurprisingly, it emerged that they had psychosocially constructed the meaning of 'deafness as a difference' in their marriage to be a 'shared burden'. Although Mike may have lacked understanding on the emotional level of the experience of deafness (Jones, Kyle and Wood, 1987), he was alongside Joy on the intellectual and practical levels. For example, he studied all aspects of Joy's original illness and was knowledgeable about the technical aspects of her cochlear implant. Furthermore, Mike supported Joy through a difficult 'tribunal' which occurred when she was unfairly dismissed from her job in a school kitchen. He also developed a specialized 'buffer' function which the literature calls 'stigma management' (Wax, 1989) when they were on holiday.

The buffer function was used with strangers, but also with members of the family. Although Sarah described herself as being 'a buffer', the role of 'mediator' is perhaps a more accurate description of her behaviour. She recalled:

> If it wasn't for me being a buffer [mediator] and saying to Joe 'This is what [my grandsons] did say'; or saying to the boys, 'This is what Grandpa heard', we would be in terrible trouble.

Gwen's mother, Beatrice, also had a mediator role. She recalled:

> [Being accepting of the difficulties presented by Arthur and Gwen's relation-
> ship] is not ... always easy. There are times when I could scream ... but I have
> coached myself ... to be [the] person in the family who tries to keep the peace.

Anthony's mother had held a similar mediating role in Clare and
Anthony's life, but she had been left behind in Nigeria. This meant that
they were left to their own devices in the continuing work of sorting out
the meaning of Anthony's deafness and the other losses in their lives.

The next section will focus on the three couples in the study who
were suddenly deafened after their marriages began, and the extra
pressures on their relationships which resulted.

Life for the newly deafened and their spouses

People experiencing a sudden profound or total loss are subject to an
instant disruption of their daily lives often accompanied by a period
of hospitalization (Ashley, 1985; Wright, 1990). This disruption
along with the inability to hear is likely to cause traumatic stress and
disorientation.

In July 1983 Anthony sustained near total deafness resulting from
drug toxicity. He was 31 years old, four years into his marriage with
Clare and the father of three young children. The event of his deafness resulted in a major domestic upheaval and crisis. In order for a
comprehensive rehabilitation programme to be implemented,
Anthony and Clare not only had to move house, they also had to
migrate to England from Nigeria where there were no rehabilitation
facilities for adults. Clare reflected that she only gradually compre-
hended how Anthony's deafness impinged on their lives:

> [Anthony] was deaf for so many years until one day he was at home, and I
> wanted to phone him from work and I suddenly realized if I phoned, he
> wouldn't hear ,... it took me some time to make [the connection in my mind].

All aspects of communication had to be examined. Anthony was also
prepared to acknowledge the problematic side of deafness especially
regarding his retraining. He wrote:

> I have to learn all my facts by reading them. A lecture of one hour can cover the
> facts in a textbook, but it takes me a week to read [the same book] ... But

because of my interest and God given ability, I [am able] to work hard, ... [and] keep abreast with hearing colleagues.

One of Anthony and Clare's major resources was their couple relationship. Because they were both Nigerian, they could act as psychosocial buffers, protecting each other from too sharp a discrepancy between inner and outer worlds (Huntingdon, 1982). In an alien environment, their culture was embodied by and in each other as well as in the Nigerian relations and friends in their social network. In this they contrasted with another couple in the study, American Rachel and British Richard. Much distress was caused in this relationship because the British spouse was seen to embody rather than buffer the foreignness of the environment.

Clare and Anthony were also aware that simply coping wasn't enough. They had to be openly positive in their outlook if they wished for the patronage and interest of white English hearing people; and, if they wished to keep the good will of their Nigerian medical friends. Therefore, they chose to perceive Anthony's deafness as a 'blessing but sometimes problematic'. This was because it had triggered the realization of their dream of migrating to England so that Anthony could retrain as a pathologist. Formerly the move had been blocked by Anthony's medical superiors in Nigeria. This positive attitude of 'acceptance' came naturally within the context of their strong Christian faith. Clare explained:

[Anthony's deafness is not] a [big] problem with us ... because our African or Christian philosophy is different, ... it does not look at deafness as ... a stumbling block to achieving objectives in life, .. in fact deafness has brought us more blessings than anything else ...

While Clare tended to see Anthony's deafness in spiritual terms, Anthony's metaphors suggested a brave doctor/soldier self-image. He said:

I never took deafness lying down. I was still aiming at the top. But many or most deaf people tend to become withdrawn ... so it discourages even the kindest helpers ... [as dependency is feared] ... In my own case, I was succeeding ... [everything] I touched turned to gold! ... so my helpers stuck by me.

Anthony backed his conscientiousness and enthusiasm with shrewd common sense. In the next section, caring roles will be revisited in the context of marriage where there is a deafened partner.

Caring roles revisited

While this mostly positive 'public account'(Cornwell, 1984) was sincere as well as shrewd, Anthony and Clare admitted that some problems connected with Anthony's deafness were difficult. At one point Clare appeared to recapitulate by calling Anthony's deafness 'the biggest problem we have ever had', a reflection of her ambivalence as she struggled with her own sense of 'loss' and isolation (Marris, 1986), specifically in her role of interpreter and monitor of Anthony's progress. It was obvious that Clare felt completely unprepared for these roles and that it had been forced upon her by circumstances. Although Clare was happy to be living in the UK, she and Anthony suffered from culture shock. Clare discussed how she prompted Anthony to speak more clearly, not only because he was deaf, but also because he was Nigerian.

> I have developed [the habit] unconsciously [of asking Anthony to clarify what he says] ... because some of the phrases he uses while they might be clear to a Nigerian, they're not so clear to a white person ... I tell him to explain more ...

While Clare discovered she had intellectual and spiritual resources to help Anthony, she also found support at the Link Centre for Deafened People in Eastbourne. She recalled:

> [The course] showed us ... the problems that deaf people face which we had been hearing [about], but didn't understand. They gave a talk about tinnitus, ... they taught us about finger spelling, ... lip-reading, ... but the most useful talk was the technique of communication, ... skills you need to do to help deaf persons communicate better ...

Anthony also spoke highly of the course, especially the practical and career advice given, and meeting other deafened people. He recalled:

> you discover that there are so many other people in your condition, you don't feel so bad again.

While the LINK course was a valuable experience, it was, nevertheless, limited. Clare and Anthony were expected to get on with the process of integrating Anthony's deafness into their daily lives which resulted in some difficult moments. Voice control was a particular concern especially in a noisy environment. Clare spoke to Anthony:

> Sometimes when we have friends [over] and you are ... [talking excitedly], ... you [start] shouting ... And sometimes [your] voice goes low, and [I] ... have to strain ... myself to hear ... [It may be] the TV's [on] too loud and that's why [I] ... can't hear ... If ... [I] tell [you ... your voice is] too low, ... [you'd] think ... [I'm criticizing you unjustly].

Anthony acknowledged the truth of Clare's analysis:

> Sometimes I take ... [Clare's monitoring] honestly, and sometimes I feel offended ... so I find it difficult.

Anthony's medical training had inadvertently prepared him for some of the problems he experienced. Clare's monitoring role was a very delicate matter for which he felt less prepared. Noise monitoring also took place in Julia and Sam's relationship. While generally a quieter person than Julia, Sam reflected:

> I think perhaps I'm a noisy person as well. [Julia] can hear anything: Bang!, Bang!, Bang! When I eat ... my jaw makes a cracking noise ... so I've had to ... make adjustments ... because it drives [Julia] crazy!

Sam's awareness illustrated how people who do not hear are able to take responsibility for the irritating noises that they sometimes make. In contrast, Anthony demanded Clare's help in monitoring his extraneous noises even though he could no longer hear them. He explained:

> I am a very sensitive person when it comes to noise. I don't like noise ... anywhere ... There are little noises I make which I don't know I'm making ... I usually find that when I eat I make a noise.

Although Clare did not share Anthony's sensitivity towards noise, she knew he needed to be followed in his efforts to form a synthesis of his hearing and deaf selves. Clare recalled:

> sometimes [I think] 'why are you making so much noise over stirring ... [the] sugar in your tea?' ... [you don't] know [you're] ... doing it so I can't tell [you] to stop because it is too much to expect of [you] ...

Clare's growing compassion for Anthony was nurtured by each new experience as she watched him struggle to do his best, constrained by deafness. While Clare's easy going attitude towards the noise made by their three children may well have been appropriate, Anthony expected her to be more vigilant as he would have been if he were hearing. Anthony complained:

> you see if the children are making noise, ... [Clare] will keep quiet, ... but my friends when they come here, they tell me that my children are very noisy ... If I could hear, my children would not make a noise.

Clare defended her assessment of the situation:

> The children don't make unnecessary noise ... [while] it looks like a lot of noise (e.g. jumping off furniture), it's normal children's noises ... the only visitors [who have] complained [are] childless, ... childless ... they don't know what it's like.

Thus parenting could become complicated when the father in his role of disciplinarian (Marsh, 1987), could not hear. Joe and Sarah also talked repeatedly about difficulties resulting from noise. Unlike Anthony, Joe could hear sound, but the sound he heard was often too loud (Gilmore, 1982). He said:

> I mean I get ... [noise from children] all the time in the summer ... I've got a place of business. There's a school about 150 yards down the road ... and they've got their own playground, and when they come out, they're shrieking and I either have to turn my hearing aids down or shut the windows.

While children's noises did not hurt Anthony in this way, Anthony's inability to trust his ears tended to spread to distrusting his wife's judgement more generally. Their associates sometimes appeared to exploit this situation. Clare admitted to feeling particularly upset at times. She recalled:

> If somebody says something, ... and I'm trying to relate [to Anthony] what the person is saying, ... [and] it's not quite exactly what he wants to hear, ... [then] he blames me, ... even though I'm trying to be helpful, ... and that's what I sometimes find annoying ... some people use me as a scapegoat.

Clare was understandably aggrieved when her efforts were misconstrued. It was likely that part of Anthony must have on occasion felt scapegoated himself, wondering why he was the one to be singled out for deafness.

The fear that one partner would 'get the wrong end of the stick' was a difficulty often mentioned. This was not to say that this was not a common occurrence among hearing couples and Clare admitted that she also 'misheard' in this way. However, deafness appeared to exacerbate the situation.

Undoubtedly when one partner has sustained sudden deafness, the couple has an immensely painful adjustment to make. The sudden loss of hearing has to be gradually accepted by both partners if the marriage is to proceed. Because of the complexities involved, it is a difficult and stressful undertaking and resembles a joint bereavement as the loss of a hearing identity is integrated into every day life experiences. The three couples in the study who were most affected by sudden deafness, Mike and Joy, Anthony and Clare, Robert and Mary, were able to overcome the potentially tragic aspect of the situation and psychosocially constructed 'deafness as a difference' respectively as 'a burden to be shared', 'a blessing, but sometimes problematic' and 'a challenging problem'.

Anthony and Clare's story was of particular interest because of the juxtaposition of the experience of sudden deafness with sudden migration and racism. All three experiences required a massive reordering to take place in their outer and inner worlds (Huntingdon, 1984).

Thoughtful reflection about present experiences so that appropriate new identities could be forged, a process for which Anthony and Clare did not always have the energy, was continually necessary to avoid embarrassment. Clare acknowledged the difficulties by relating one example. She felt deep embarrassment that Anthony no longer spoke his native 'Ibo' when meeting members of his tribe in the UK. Although Clare did not say so explicitly, perhaps Anthony did not currently have the confidence that he could successfully lipread Ibo; and therefore spoke English, the language of the country which had 'adopted' him in his need for rehabilitation.

For the marriage to survive, hearing partners discovered that they became the front line, informal, full-time rehabilitators as acceptance and integration began and progressed. They had to find the emotional strength to contain their partners as they struggled to synthesize the deaf and hearing parts of themselves. In this respect their experiences resembled the children of deaf parents (Preston, 1994). For example, Anthony wished to hang on to his sensitivity to noises from his 'hearing self', even though his new 'deaf self' could not actually hear them. In a similar way, Joy wished to hang on to all the friendships which she had made when she was hearing although her deaf self could not have intimate chats with them on the telephone. Similarly, Joe prided himself on coming from a musical family and delighted in his record collection although what he actually heard was bound to be affected by the inevitable distortion which still exists in hearing aid amplification. It was these threads of continuity which interwove to bring back a sense of normality and well being into the lives of the deafened people in this study.

Some spouses refused to provide the demanding support needed at the time a profound hearing loss was acknowledged and their marriages fell apart. Their stories will be discussed at the end of this chapter.

The couples discussed so far had sustained severe, profound or total losses of hearing. We will now examine the three couples in the study where one partner gradually acquired their hearing loss which was of a mild/moderate degree.

Mild and recent hearing loss

Anne and Adam

The literature (Cowrie and Douglas-Cowrie), suggests that people with mild/moderate hearing loss are likely to be better adjusted than individuals with more severe hearing loss. Findings emerging from this study proved the situation to be more complex.

Anne, a social researcher, recalled how her husband Adam, an education manager, encouraged her to have her hearing tested as he had noticed she didn't always hear him. After seeing the Audiologist who confirmed her mild/moderate loss, she reflected:

> but having been [diagnosed], I feel I have labelled myself.

Having a 'label' made Anne feel odd and different in a way she disliked. She was also very unsure of the implications:

> For example ... our car insurance ... says 'have you got any disability?' Because in a sense I have because it has been 'labelled' [but I also feel that] I don't want to draw attention to anything ... it's not significant enough.

Adam added:

> The most pronounced situation ... [was] in the countryside in the summer ... and the crickets were making a lot of noise and everybody could hear them [but] ... Anne.

Anne had a different opinion:

> When I think about [people saying] there are crickets going, ... [I think] other people are [just] imagining things ... it was a holiday ... it was outside of every-day reality.

Anne was beginning to manage her hearing loss and she refused to become distressed about not hearing things which she saw as unimportant to the main thrust of her life and interests. However, music was a different matter. She recalled:

> just before Christmas, we went to a concert, and there I suddenly thought, ... 'Am I going to miss some of the higher notes?', .. .and that I would mind a lot, ... but it was fine ... [the music] sounded the same as usual.

Anne wished to test different situations to see how they were affected by a high frequency hearing loss. Adam thought Anne was not fully comprehending the difficulties ahead. He recalled:

> [Recently) ... I ... [went] to dinner with some [African] ... students, and their accents are very broad and very difficult for me to understand ... I am certain that Anne would have been totally lost.

Anne disagreed with Adam's specific point, but thought he might be correct in principle as she had not been able to hear one of her students with a strong Welsh accent.

Once Anne had thoughtfully assessed the situation, she and Adam perceived the meaning of 'deafness as a difference' within their relationship as 'a problem to be watched'.

Frank and Simone

Frank, an academic administrator, also had a mild/moderate hearing loss. Unlike Anne, it had not been a surprise as mild deafness had been in the family. He recalled:

> my grandmother ... [and] mother [were also] deaf, but neither of my sisters or ... other brother ... [are], a lot is hereditary ... it's ... the chance factor ... I've just got to accept ... that there are certain things I won't be able to hear.

Although Frank sounded stoical in his acceptance of his hearing problem, he appeared to need reassurance that he hadn't been singled out for some special punishment which his brother and sisters had escaped. Because he was both gifted and fortunate in both career and family life, his hearing loss appeared to represent 'an occasional source of sadness', something he didn't quite know how to address since it didn't fit in with his otherwise almost golden existence and well deserved achievements. Frank revealed how he managed these feelings:

> there are times when I haven't heard something and I should have heard it and I've said [to myself] 'Oh, I feel sorry that I haven't heard it' and in that sense I feel a bit frustrated ... on the other hand, what's the point of being frustrated all the time? ... it won't help me ...

Frank explained further how he had learned to cope:

> I suppose I go quiet. I mean my sister said to me, 'Were you all right on Saturday [night at my dinner party] because you were very quiet?' and I said, 'Well, I just couldn't compete'.

While Frank put his withdrawal down to his deafness, his wife Simone, disagreed for she said:

> but I feel it was the same before you became deaf ... Frank would go quiet before the loss of hearing because [that's his) personality.

Frank acknowledged her point saying:

> I don't like ... situations in which a lot of people are trying to dominate, ... I like a give and take situation in which people make a point ... [then] other people might respond to that one.

Like Anne, Frank found some situations difficult and sought to maintain a sense of personal control by deciding whether or not a given conversation was important enough to ask for clarification. This capacity for discrimination had been acquired by both of them before becoming hearing impaired, but now it had an additional function. Anne and Frank's hearing partners, however, did not see their partner's withdrawal in social situations in the same positive light.

Rachel and Richard

American Rachel and British Richard were the only couple in the study to contain a conductive hearing loss, otosclerosis, within their relationship. This condition involves the deterioration of small bones in the middle ear. Otosclerosis is unlike sensorineural hearing loss in that it will respond to microsurgery. Rachel had one operation which was successful initially; but over time after the birth of her two sons, the condition re-emerged.

Rachel and Richard are the only couple in this book who openly acknowledged having a communication problem in their marriage for which they had sought professional help. Although Rachel's deafness may have exacerbated their marital troubles, neither partner saw it as doing so as hearing aid distortion does not occur in the same way with a conductive loss as happens in a sensorineural loss. Rachel and Richard had psychosocially constructed 'deafness as a difference' to mean 'a nuisance'. She revealed this attitude when describing how she felt about the possibility of not having to wear hearing aids. She said:

> I was very excited to think that without aids, I could go swimming, you know ... could run around, ... outside they whistle ... yes, yes, they're a nuisance ... [How I would] love to get rid of these awful things.

It appeared to be the wearing of the aids rather than her deafness as such which Rachel allowed to inhibit her from doing some of her favourite activities. This is puzzling as it is quite possible to swim without them, but only if one is comfortable with not hearing.

In comparing a mild loss with the experience of sudden deafness, there were fewer difficulties with which to come to terms, as communication and identity were not as severely affected. For example, there was no need for assistive aids except the hearing aid on occasion, and there was no pressure on the hearing spouse to carry a rehabilitator's role, although some 'awareness' was felt to be helpful. This was not to suggest that a mild/moderate hearing loss was insignificant as it had the tendency to spoil 'the perfect', especially for men who have been socialized to connect their feeling of manliness with being physically a 'complete man' (Stevens, 1966). A mild/moderate hearing loss had to be thought about and managed by various coping strategies meaning that some understanding and appropriate sympathy was appreciated. However, the latter was rarely asked for or rarely received, meaning that there is something especially isolating about having a mild/moderate hearing loss.

Summary

In this chapter, the Epigenetic principle has been used for looking at the ways in which hearing loss affects couples in the basic process of attachment/care giving. The couples concerned were significantly different from those in Parker's study in their coping patterns, although there were also similarities especially during the time immediately following the onset of sudden deafness. In such circumstances, both studies revealed that it was 'the quality' of the marriage which determined whether or not it held together.

If the marriages were to move forward, the couples needed to agree on a way to perceive the deafness within their relationships. The three couples in this study where one partner was suddenly deafened described the deafness as 'a blessing, but sometimes problematic', 'a shared burden', and 'a challenging problem'. The three couples where one partner had acquired a mild/moderate loss described it as 'a problem to be watched', 'an occasional source of sadness', and 'a nuisance'.

In doing so, the couples continued the behaviour first presented in Chapter 4 by focusing on 'differences' as part of an anthropological/cultural model rather than on a medical model. If this did not produce a new equilibrium, the initial commitment dissolved as occurred with four couples in this study. Their stories were told to illuminate some of the factors which cause marriage breakdown, and the specific place of hearing impairment. It emerged that deafness was an exacerbating factor to the breakdowns and one of many differences which the partners had difficulty managing.

In the context of a renegotiated contract, it is possible for 'care' to be interpreted as 'the roles' occasionally adopted by the hearing partner on behalf of the hearing impaired partner. For example, the roles which emerged were buffer, interpreter (interpreting on the telephone was considered the most stressful), mediator, prompter, advocate, and editor.

There are, however, a number of difficulties in making this connection. Firstly, the help provided by the able bodied partner, specifically the hearing spouse for the hearing impaired spouse, rarely caused the distress found by Ungerson (1987) and Parker (1993); although in certain specific situations, the findings suggested that stress, frustration and resentment were caused. In acknowledging this, it needs to be remembered that stress, frustration and resentment occur in every close relationship as these feelings are a part of human nature. Many would argue that the institution of marriage itself brings about negative feelings to an extreme degree as partially evidenced by the high divorce rate. Secondly, care was rarely provided on a daily basis, but only occasionally when needed for specific events. Thirdly, the hearing impaired member of every couple was employed in a paid or volunteer capacity, and able to function in the public sphere completely independently from their partner. Finally in focusing on this kind of 'care', it is not being suggested that the relationship was not reciprocal in the long term. On the contrary, a loving rapport on both sides seemed one of the most significant and striking features of most of the study couples. However, initially, it was not always evident how the eight people with the more severe/profound losses in the study returned the social access support that was so obviously and generously given.

The couple Anthony and Clare were chosen as a special illustration since besides sudden deafness, they also had to come to terms with sudden racism and migration. All three experiences involve a loss or change of identity in the present and the need to work towards a reintegration of what has been lost so that a reinvestment in the future may be made.

The loss of spontaneity within their couple relationship emerged as hearing partners' most frequent complaint. As often as this disappointment was acknowledged, it was also observed that there were other psychosocial factors which contributed to a more serious attitude within the marriage, for example growing older, personality traits, migration/racial issues, and other problems and responsibilities. It was exceedingly difficult to distinguish when a problem was the impact of hearing impairment, another factor, or a combination of factors of which hearing impairment was one.

In the following chapter we complete our examination of the couples in the study focusing on the three more advanced relational processes suggested by the Epigenetic framework: communication, problem-solving and mutuality or the evolving couple.

CHAPTER 6

Evolving couple relationships

Introduction

This chapter revisits all the people in the study, those with and without partners, and further develops the analysis continuing to use the Epigenetic Principle. While Chapter 5 examined the basic process of attachment/caregiving, here the focus is on the advanced processes of communication, problem-solving and mutuality. This latter process of mutuality is, in fact, found to have the most relevance for this study. Four sub-processes emerge here. They are distance management and cohesion, adaptability and change, patterns of leisure and breakdown of intimacy. First, a short theoretical review of each process as it is analysed.

Second relational process : communication

'Communication' following attachment/care giving in the Epigenetic Schema is a symbolic, transactional process or the process of creating shared meanings (Bowlby, 1975). Words or verbal behaviour are the most commonly used symbols, but a whole range of nonverbal behaviour is also included. To say that communication is transactional is to say that the participants have a mutual impact upon each other.

A transactional view of communication and a systems perspective complement each other because they both focus on relationships. In other words, relationships take precedence over individuals. As two people interact, each creates a context for the other and relates to the other within that context (Galvin and Brommel, 1991).

Communication and gender

People in the study appeared to hold certain implicit assumptions about how women and men communicate as documented in the literature by sociologists (Komarovsky, 1962), psychologists, and linguists (Tannen, 1991). Sam, Joe, Adam and Frank liked to give the impression that 'women's talk' wasn't worth listening to, a defence often used by hearing impaired men. However, gender is only one of a number of factors that seemed to influence communication in this study. Certain basic conditions were needed which will be discussed in the next section.

Communication and conflict with reference to time and place

The 'time' and 'place' of conversations were mentioned by a number of people in the study as significant in determining the effectiveness of communication. For example, Sam and Julia discovered that the best place for a conversation was in bed where they could relax, while Joe and Sarah felt the best time to talk was on Saturday mornings when they didn't have to rush off to work. Couples also had their worst places for communication. Hearing Julia acknowledged that she had the greatest difficulty hearing Sam in pubs and in the street. Because Sam was unable to hear the volume of his own voice, he sometimes spoke exceptionally softly in these places. Clare has already introduced us to this phenomenon which occurred occasionally in her conversations with Anthony. Barbara and Ben and Joy and Mike talked about their communication difficulties when driving in a car after dark. The most difficult places for Joe and Frank were in the street or on public transport. Joe related:

> [when] we go on a bus [or a train], [Sarah and I will] sit together ... quietly, travelling where we are going, ... and say nothing ...

Psychological and emotional factors also played a part in whether or not communication was effective such as the presence or absence of feelings of anger and hostility. Sometimes these negative feelings combined with hearing loss to cause conflict as Adam explained:

> Sometimes ... [Anne] will get irritated with me because she has asked me something [and] ... I've replied, ... but she hasn't heard [my response], ... and she will then raise her voice in a slightly irritable way ... [Although I have replied to her], she will shout at me ...

Anne defended herself:

> I don't shout at you ... it's to do with the feeling that [Adam] is not very communicative, ... so if I feel I've said something that hasn't brought a response, ... the meaning [to me] ... is that he is not communicating.

This was an excellent example of how a relatively mild hearing loss could cause misunderstandings and exacerbates the difficulties in communication which were already present.

Communication and lip-reading

The study produced a wealth of information on this topic. Five areas of lip-reading stress were investigated. They were when encountering strangers, when intimacy is lost with children, the gender factor, within committed partnerships, and fear of intimacy. Further details can be found in two articles (Morgan-Jones, 1993, 1998).

The next section will look at joint problem-solving, the third relational process in Wynne's schema.

Third relational process: joint problem-solving

When the processes of attachment/care giving and communication have been relatively successful, they lead to the next relational process of joint problem-solving. If communication has previously been dysfunctional, bogged down, or distorted by enmeshment or disengagement, this fact is most likely to emerge during the problem-solving stage.

Joint problem-solving was a difficult area to explore with the study couples because the partners appeared at times to have difficulty in identifying what was 'a joint problem'. This meant that one partner would identify a problem that concerned them, sometimes connected with hearing loss and sometimes not, while the other partner would attempt to understand the reasons for their concern.

For example, deafened Joy and hearing Mary both found it problematic when their husbands engaged in great arguments with their grown up sons especially as visits from these sons were rare. The husbands, Mike and Robert, did not understand why their behaviour was problematic as it felt 'fine' to them. Two spouses, Frank and Rachel found problematic the way in which their partners expressed themselves. Frank felt his French wife expressed herself too dramatically resulting in his feeling berated at times, while Rachel felt her husband was under expressive resulting in her feeling taken for granted.

In a similar way, problems more directly connected with hearing impairment were not jointly experienced. For example, it was difficult for Ben to understand how frustrating it was for hearing impaired Barbara not to have 'subtitles' for the television; it was difficult for Clare to understand fully how annoying the children's noise level was for deafened Anthony; it was difficult for Kay to understand what a strain it was for hearing impaired Henry when he could not relate to people properly during the noisy fellowship hour after church. Conversely, it was hard for hearing impaired Joe to understand how difficult it was for Sarah when she tried to help him while out shopping, or for hearing impaired Joy to understand how frustrating it was for Mike when he tried to balance his own needs with that of his wife's in social situations.

However, once a problem was identified and jointly accepted as such, the couples had no difficulty in working through the other steps. For example, Sarah and Joe identified the 'loss' of his two sons by his first marriage as a tragic problem. After a twenty year gap, Joe's sons were eventually contacted, welcomed into their home, and reunited with their father. Frank and Simone had agreed earlier in their marriage that the 'night terrors' of their twins were a problem, and Robert and Mary agreed that the emotional breakdown of their youngest adult son was a problem. In both families, the parents took steps to support their children through these critical times.

Thus the couples had no difficulty in joint problem-solving once the problem was jointly identified. This suggests that counselling work with couples where one partner is hearing impaired may need to focus on the identification and mutual acceptance of joint problems initially, and only later to focus on the solving process itself.

The next section will look at mutuality, the fourth process which enfolds epigenetically in relational systems.

Fourth relational process: mutuality

The central aspect of 'mutuality' is that the partners have a shared commitment to one another to shape their relationship as the life-cycle unfolds, as expected and unexpected events occur, and as new tasks and aspirations emerge. Mutuality also incorporates a selective integration of the preceding processes of attachment/care giving, communication, and joint problem-solving; and thus draws upon the acquired relational experience and skill which has emerged from each of these prior stages.

The four aspects of mutuality which will be explored in the next section are distance management/cohesion, adaptability/change, leisure patterns, and the breakdown of intimacy. It needs to be recalled that distance management/cohesion and adaptability are two of the family dimensions identified by Olson *et al.* (1983) in formulating the circumplex model of marital and family systems. Here they are discussed under the heading of 'mutuality'.

Distance management and cohesion

Study couples managed their need for closeness and distance in various ways. Sarah, wife of severely hearing impaired Joe, feared too much time in his company would render her incapable of spontaneous conversation. She recalled:

> But sometimes I just think I become very quiet, and of course when I meet other people, I have stopped talking haven't I?

Sarah's 'drying up syndrome' was not just a response to Joe's deafness, it was also a response to 'the differences' between people which are found in all intimate relationships. While Sarah knew the importance of social support networks to compensate for differences, some study couples were not interested in making such efforts, but preferred to lose themselves in reading, a good hobby or project, or simply time on one's own. Henry explained:

> When I'm studying, I take my hearing aids off my glasses and try to lose myself in what I'm doing, ... so I'm escaping from the hearing world ... [In this way, the outside of myself and] the inside [are] in tune with what I'm doing ... [with no disturbing background noises].

Henry recreated his sense of well being, sometimes diminished in the 'hearing world', by concentration and total emersion in his studies.

Byng-Hall (1985) suggests that all partners, regardless of hearing ability, need time for escaping from their marriage. Hearing Sarah, in making an issue of her need for distance management from Joe, had lost sight of the anthropological approach (Preston, 1994). However, she regained it again when she focused on Joe's helpfulness:

> Joe listens and he's very good ... the trouble is I have all the energy [to share my problems] at a quarter to eight in the morning when I need to be getting to work!

Sarah pointed to the pressures of 'time' and 'place' as inhibiting factors in this kind of intimate dialogue. Sarah recounted a recent experience on holiday with Joe:

> We ... wanted one week away without ... [distractions] ... I want[ed] to ... talk to my husband, and for him to listen to me ... we went and we got food, and we cooked it 'at home' so we could talk over our meals, ... and we [had a wonderful time catching] up on things.

Although Joe might not have a talent for 'small talk', he was more than capable of being a good companion and participating in more advanced relational processes, specifically intimacy and communication.

Adaptability and change

Olson and McCubbin describe adaptability as being 'the ability of a marital/family system to change its power structure, role relationships, and relationship rules in response to situation and developmental stress' (Olson *et al.*, 1983: 62).

Managing roles may become more complex when marriages must also cope with a disability. Role shifts or reversals sometimes take place that put extra strain on marriages (Hoad, Oliver and

Silver, 1990). Oliver (1983) mentions difficulties with 'role overload' while House and Robbins (1983) mention 'role strain'.

The people in this book did not appear to have any special difficulties in managing household chores with respect to their disability. Specific difficulties were mentioned only once by the retired couple, Mary and Robert. Robert had troubles with decorating, heavy lifting, and cleaning, jobs he had done before he contracted Menière's Disease. As a practical person, Mary did not resent Robert's withdrawal from these areas for she saw he was much happier absorbed in his writing and volunteer activities. Of the ten remaining couples, eight out of ten women, regardless of hearing ability, took the major responsibility for looking after the household. Husbands generally saw themselves as helpers or 'understudies' as described by Rapoport and Rapoport (1971). The two remaining men, Ben and Joe, took on more responsibility for family/household management as their wives considered most chores boring and preferred to focus their energies elsewhere. Joy was also in this group and it was hoped that a more balanced distribution of chores would occur after Mike retired. Four people in the study had hired help. Anne, Sarah, and Simone had weekly cleaning ladies and Rachel and Richard hired a monthly gardener.

Traditional gender roles appeared to be barely affected by one partner having a hearing loss. Other contributory psychosocial factors were personal inclination, convenience, talents, and skills. A high degree of 'adaptability' was noted (Olson *et al.*, 1983) in that the partners relied on each other both to support and to counterbalance each others' movements (Clulow and Mattinson, 1989).

For example, all the men, whether hearing or hearing impaired, could look after themselves if their wives were away. Most of them had specific cooking skills and exercised them from time to time such as making breakfast, curries, casseroles, cooking with a wok, or making wine. There was a general feeling among the couples specifically Anthony and Clare, Ben and Barbara, Henry and Kay, Joe and Sarah, that they made a successful team. This was particularly true in such tasks as entertaining, planning for a foreign holiday, and decorating.

Patterns of leisure

Changing patterns of leisure was a challenging factor mentioned by couples where deafness struck after their marriage was established.

Couples who had once enjoyed the theatre, the cinema, and dancing no longer received the same mutual enjoyment and stimulus which they once had done. Deafened Joy recalled:

> With dancing, I think ... to a certain extent it is pointless [because I can't hear the music] ... There is some enjoyment ... obviously ...

Despite the difficulties, Mike and Joy often choose holiday resorts where they could dance. Mike said:

> I mean ... [Joy] does get up on the floor at modern disco dancing ... even if she's never heard disco music ... [before]! ...

Joy's inability to hear the music did not prevent her from responding to Mike's enthusiasms. Later Mike revealed that they had actually won a dance prize. He explained:

> Joy does follow ... we don't make mistakes ... I can still enjoy the music and the dancing at the same time ... we won a dancing competition on holiday a couple of years ago.

Joy acknowledged her ability to follow:

> I sort of have a vague idea of music in my ... [head]. I'm used to dancing with Mike and follow him easily, [and] I can follow other people.

Along with following, there was a hint of skill. Joy also admitted that she was able to experience some enjoyment from the general atmosphere:

> it's not the same as being able to hear, ... but to a certain extent you pick up the [atmosphere] ... you more or less make yourself join in.

Because Joy knew that Mike would give up the dancing he loved if she did not go too, she tagged along in an effort to bring him happiness. Thus she was willing to compromise since she knew that in other areas it was Mike who did the compromising.

Deafened Anthony, severely deaf Henry, and prelingually deaf Arthur all admitted that they had almost no leisure time with their wives. As all three were involved in serious courses of study, it was hoped that the situation would change after they completed their degrees.

Couples who met when one partner was already hearing impaired seemed to have fewer regrets with respect to leisure activities. From the beginning certain activities were established as ones which they enjoyed doing together while others were off limits. In the case of Barbara and Ben, a day out together meant attending a Lautrec exhibition or a visit to Hatchard's bookshop. Julia and Sam were both sporty and enjoyed a good tennis match or a walk in the country while Sarah and Joe enjoyed going on holidays to unknown parts.

The general pattern of couple leisure that emerged was a varied one. Some activities stopped, others were altered or restructured, and still others continued with little change. This did not seem significantly different from couples where both partners could hear as their leisure interests change and develop over the life-cycle (Rapoport and Rapoport, 1975). What was likely to be different was the criteria used when making decisions about leisure activities. That is, would a hearing loss be an obstacle to enjoyment?

We now consider what happens when couples lack the wisdom, love, or skill to manage 'deafness as a difference' or other difficulties within their marriage.

Breakdown of intimacy

One of the most significant social trends in post war Britain has been the steady escalation of marital breakdown (Clark and Haldane, 1990). People's behaviour in this study reflected the national trends. It emerged that one quarter of the study couples had experienced marital breakdown including one couple who divorced after the interviewing was complete. Although this figure roughly suggests that hearing couples have a higher chance of divorce than when one partner has a hearing loss, the situation is more complex. A brief analysis of the marriages that ended suggested a number of common factors.

A factor which united the four couples was that they were all in Stage IV in the family life-cycle, sometimes called the Stage of Adolescence when their marriages dissolved. It is a time when marital satisfaction is likely to be the lowest and stress the highest (Bernard, 1982). The divorcing study couples had succeeded in getting beyond the average time of divorce for hearing couples of between five and nine years after the wedding (One Plus One, 1998); but had run in to trouble in the early part of their third marital decade: 20, 21, 22 and 24 years of marriage respectively.

The four divorcing couples in this study were placed in three groups. Two women, Christine and Grace, formed the first group. Although they had both grown up knowing they were hearing impaired, as high spirited women, it had not held them back from personal, artistic, and academic achievements. Grace was an interior decorator and refurbisher while Christine was a gifted musician and counsellor. However, Christine now 70, a retired rehabilitation counsellor, recalled her confused feelings before she married Jack:

> [Jack and I] talked to each other ... [a little about my hearing loss], ... I was still going through a 'denial' period ... I remember thinking as [Jack and I] were driving off after Church, 'Why are you going to marry me? ... I'll probably be stone-deaf before anything ... no I can't [tell you] that' ... I wanted to marry Jack, I wanted to have a family, I wanted to have a normal existence and for twenty-five years I did.

Christine decided to a adopt a 'pretence' strategy (Higgens, 1980). Both she and Grace married high-achieving verbal men and delighted in the role of 'helpmate'. Christine had three children and became the ideal doctor's wife. In hindsight, she wished she had been more honest with her boys. She recalled:

> If I had it to do over again, I would be much more open about [being hearing impaired]. I ... [didn't] want to burden my family with my troubles, and if I could work around it, I would ...

Christine's 'denial' of her deafness protected her family and herself from the reality of her growing isolation. Her attitude was similar to Barbara's and Ben's since they also wished to retain their children's innocence (see Chapter 7). While Christine immersed herself in family life, Grace and her husband, George, did not have children. Grace preferred to support their joint business by making good use of her contacts with 'dealers' and her flair in discovering tasteful bargains.

A psychological phenomenon called a 'critical mass' (Wax, 1989) was formed . This precipitated in the breaking down of Christine's and Grace's partnerships and their 'pretence strategies' (Higgens, 1980). Grace recalled:

> As far as husbands and wives are concerned, my private opinion is that [their happiness together] ... depends on what sort of social position they have. After all, some people don't expect anything in the sense of a social life, even when they can hear. Their social life is very small. Whereas the higher on the social scale you go, the more you expect such as sophisticated dinner parties. My deafness put a 'lid' on this. My ex-husband, who is a great conversationalist, ... said he could not see why he had to suffer too.

As Grace and George had built their marriage around a 'business and social partnership', the marriage ended when Grace could no longer keep up with her husband's social verbosity. George's so called 'commitment' had apparently lacked the deeper roots of true emotional intimacy or an emotional 'couple fit' which could sustain an acceptance of 'loss' as part of the human condition (Morgan-Jones, 1991).

Christine and Jack's relationship was also built on the assumption of perfect hearing. When the 'denial' was broken and reality revealed, Jack's feelings of commitment also faltered. Christine recalled:

> .he went off with another woman, ... [but] he kept coming back. He really didn't want to break up the family, but he couldn't break up with this woman either, and he died [of hepatitis] a month after the divorce was filed ...

Although Jack died at the age of 50 in a state of turmoil, Christine was now free to put her relationship with her children and grandchildren on a more honest footing, and to develop her burgeoning career. With the passing of time, Christine forgave Jack as she was aware that only as an independent woman could she have found the courage to take control of her life.

The second category was composed of Joe and his first wife, Emma. Like Christine and Grace, his marriage was dissolved, but with a different outcome (see Chapter 4). Perhaps because he was more confident than they were, he did not hide his hearing loss and could inform people of its existence. However, he was never able to communicate his 'special needs' for attention fully to his wife Emma who focused most of her time and energy on their two young sons and her plans for their brilliant careers. Resentments grew and they parted. After the death of both his parents and a period of great loneliness, Joe married Sarah.

All three stories have one point in common. The deafness itself within the relationship did not cause the break up of the marriages despite the fact that the hearing impaired partners initially told their stories to the researcher in such a way as to make it appear that it had. This is because hearing loss makes an easy 'hook' on which to blame things. When the relationships, however, were analysed, it emerged that all three couples had substantial difficulties with managing 'differences' generally with the hearing loss representing one additional 'difference'. Underdeveloped communication skills were likely to be the main reason why these couples did not manage differences appropriately.

The third category comprised Adam and Anne who divorced during the writing of this study. The relationship was significantly different from the other three couples mentioned in that the hearing loss was never an issue in the marriage, although it is possible that it was an exacerbating factor (see Chapter 9 for further examples of couples who experienced a breakdown of intimacy).

Summary

This chapter completes the use of the Epigenetic Schema in the analysis, looking this time at all the people in the study. While communication and problem-solving revealed some interesting material, the most relevant for this study were the four sub-processes which emerged: distance management and cohesion, adaptability and change, patterns of leisure and break down of intimacy. This latter section facilitated the analysis of the divorcing couples in the study. It revealed that all four couples had run into major difficulties in their third marital decade. This suggests they were able to navigate the most difficult time for hearing couples, five to nine years into the marriage when children are often small, but could not manage the Adolescent Stage, another period where marriage satisfaction is known to be low. This suggests that the extra tensions involved in beginning and establishing a family did not cause as many difficulties for the couples in this study as the tensions involved with nurturing and launching teenage children.

The point is also made that couples where one person is hearing and the other is hearing impaired have an understandable tendency to blame the hearing loss for the breakdown of their relationship. A deeper analysis suggests that a hearing loss for the study's participants who divorced was an exacerbating factor, but not the fundamental reason for the marriage break-up. While multiple factors usually contribute to marital breakdown, the couples in this study appear to have the most difficulty with underdeveloped communication skills especially in managing differences as opposed to problems with actual verbal facility, although the two problems could go together.

From the couple, the focus will now shift to the family especially the impact hearing impairment may have on children when one of their parents has a hearing impairment.

CHAPTER 7

Families and children

Introduction

Very little comprehensive research has been done into the ways children cope when one parent is hearing and the other parent has a hearing loss (SHHH, July/August, 1999). Before exploring this topic in this current study, we will explore its theoretical foundations.

The family life-cycle approach is generally associated with the developmental perspective over the life span (Duvall and Hill, 1948). It ranges from the formation to the dissolution of family units. Families are followed as they move through stages of development and the tasks associated with each. An examination is also made of the transitions between stages that punctuate the life-cycle and represent major additions, losses or modifications of roles.

This approach is not to be confused with the family life course approach which many sociological researchers in the UK prefer because it allows for more 'flexible biographical patterns within a continually changing social system' (Cohen, 1987). In this specific study, the family life-cycle approach was retained largely because the people's lives were relatively conventional in their structure, and therefore fitted the framework of the life-cycle approach. However, it needs to be clarified that an 'ideal' is not being suggested or that there is a denial of the numerous variations found in family life today (Walsh and McGoldrick, 1991; Barratte et al., 1999).

Lastly, the family life-cycle has been found useful for examining the nature of family stress, a biological and psychological reaction which may be triggered by the onset of hearing impairment in a family member. Such stressors may or may not produce a family 'crisis'. Hill defines a 'stressor' as a situation for which a family has had no preparation so that members' ability to deal with it is problematic (1949). A family 'crisis', predictable or unpredictable, is described as occurring when the family can no longer make use of its resources (for example problem-solving ability, common sense, communication patterns) in a way that 'controls and contains the forces of change' (Joselevich, 1988: 273).

In the following section, each family life stage is introduced and briefly described. Then findings related to each stage are analyzed so that the usefulness of this approach emerges.

Stage I: Young couple without children

Here the partners are adjusting to living as a committed pair. Couples without children are likely to be both flexible and cohesive in their manner of relating to one another (Olson, Lavee and McCubbin, 1988). This implies stronger external than internal boundaries, with flexible interactional rules and roles.

The study produced two couples in this stage, Arthur and Gwen and Sam and Julia. While Arthur and Gwen were newly married and were experiencing a transition as they moved from Stage I to II in that their first child, a son, was born during the interviewing period, Sam and Julia had cohabited without children for ten years. They appeared to approach their relationship in the spirit of gratitude, a reflection perhaps of the fact that both of them had experienced considerable 'loss'. Children were being considered, but a decision had not yet been made.

Stage II: Families with preschool children (aged 0–5)

At this stage the family reorganizes around the needs of the infant(s) and becomes a permanent system for the first time. This means that symbolically and in reality this transition is the key one in the family life-cycle (McGoldrick, 1991). Even with dual career couples, there is a return to more traditional sex roles usually resulting in a lowering of self-esteem for women (Cowen *et al.*, 1985) and ambivalence for men.

Severely hearing impaired Joe was the one person in the study to admit to his feelings of jealousy towards his two sons. Nevertheless, it was the birth of his eldest son that helped him towards a more realistic assessment of his hearing loss in that it prompted him to purchase his first hearing aid because 'children have soft voices'. Such remarks underline the complex and powerful nature of parental feelings, specifically fathers' towards the birth of their children (Clulow and Mattinson, 1989).

After the birth of his baby son, profoundly deaf Arthur admitted that he felt mildly excluded. His hearing wife, Gwen, had not only an infant to care for, but also a recently widowed mother.

Severely deaf Henry recalled feeling immensely proud after the birth of his son. Simultaneously, he felt somewhat envious of his wife because of the attention she received from concerned people in the community. He remembered that everyone always asked how Kay, the mother, was doing, apparently unaware how enormously involved he was as a father. Thus while Henry felt included in the family bonding taking place, he appeared to feel excluded from public recognition of the emotional and physical cost of that bonding (SSA Magazine, 1993).

Henry was also concerned about whether or not his children would inherit his deafness. Although logically he understood that his own deafness was the result of his mother having had rubella, he was relieved when their son, Clive, was tested and found to have normal hearing at the age of eight months. This had not been a concern of his hearing wife, Kay, who had long before noticed that their son was responsive to sound especially to music, and that had been enough for her.

Understandably, Henry was also anxious about whether he could lip-read Clive when he began to talk. It quickly became apparent that Clive's speech like all children's, came gradually and Henry could easily keep up with it. Henry also discovered that reading a chosen story book together at the end of the day was a good way of nurturing their relationship and his lip-reading ability as well. Playing together with Hornby trains was another favoured activity for similar reasons.

Lastly, while Henry was working out the best way to communicate with Clive, Clive discovered that his father was hearing impaired and sought to adjust his own behaviour accordingly. Between the ages of two and a half and three and a half, Clive realized that having a 'deaf' father meant that he, Clive, had to go

directly to his father if he wanted to tell him that tea was ready, and
that he would not be heard if he yelled from the bottom of the stairs.
Understanding how his father needed to lip-read, however, was a
slightly more demanding exercise. For example, Clive, would sometimes start to talk to his father when his back was turned. When Kay
noticed this, she would say to Clive:

> Daddy is not hearing you because he's not looking at you.

This helped Clive's understanding to develop on how best to
communicate with his father. Kay and Henry also recalled how
Clive would sometimes stop in the middle of a conversation at the
dinner table, and demand: 'Mummy, look at me, I'm talking to you',
or 'Daddy, look at me, I'm talking to you.'

Thus he had generalized the 'looking' behaviour to all conversations between adults and children. As he grew a little older, he was
able to discriminate that it was his father and not his mother who
needed to look in order to hear. However, he would still ask to be
looked at by his mother if she wasn't responding to his conversation
appropriately because of her other preoccupations.

Young children do need to experiment with the concept of deafness in relation to themselves. Although Leah Cohen (1994) did not
have a deaf parent, she spent her early childhood living in the midst
of deaf people at the Lexington School for the Deaf in New York
City. She recalled putting pebbles in her ears to simulate hearing aids
at the age of four. Not surprisingly, Clive also experimented by
claiming to be deaf when he didn't wish to respond to what his
mother was saying such as 'Come and wash your hands for dinner'.
Kay, concerned that Clive now thought deafness was something one
could control, tried a little 'awareness' experiment with him. At one
point, she stuck her fingers in both his ears explaining his frustration
in not being able to hear was what it was like for Daddy most of the
time. She added:

> and you [Clive] mustn't say you are deaf, because we know that you are not
> deaf.

This was rather a severe test for so small a child whose thinking is
often primitive and magical (Fraiberg, 1959). On the other hand,

Clive's responses were promising, and it was thought likely that he could cope with the lessons he was receiving since they were given simply and within a warm family atmosphere.

The above account reflects a child at this stage struggling with the meaning of deafness, a trait of his father's that required him to make certain adjustments before effective communication could take place. As he struggled with the concept of physical deafness in his father, he invariably stumbled on defensive psychological deafness in his mother and himself, namely not hearing when one was preoccupied or didn't wish to respond to what was being asked or demanded.

In comparing Henry and Kay's approach with the two couples who had latency aged children, the former were the most conscientious in their perceived responsibility to teach 'deaf awareness'. Perhaps partly because the children in the two other families were slightly older, their parents had difficulty in recalling these earlier stages. One couple, Barbara and Ben, seemed almost proud that they had taught nothing directly to their children about Barbara's severe deafness. The fact that Louise and Edward facilitated their mother's lip-reading by facing her when they spoke, was seen as having occurred naturally without prompting from adults. They believed that further disability awareness would occur when the children were ready. Consequently, Barbara was prepared to put up with demanding behaviour in the desire not to spoil Louise and Edward's childhoods as naive hearing children.

For example, while Clive was learning at age three that he needed to fetch his father rather than call him from the foot of the stairs, Louise and Edward at seven and nine years of age were still calling for their mother when they were on one level of the house and she was on the other, and getting frustrated when she did not appear. Thus, Barbara's deafness was perceived by her family as a 'frustration'. Barbara and Ben's attitude appeared to reflect the following statement found in the disability literature:

> We have to let our sons and daughters be children and do the things they want. They have their own little minds and their own priorities. We can't let them become robots for our sake (Brown, 1981: 35)

Nevertheless, making demands on children is appropriate in certain circumstances. Most small children are instinctively highly motivated to communicate with their parents verbally and nonverbally (Klein, 1987). More often than not, children are happy to place themselves in front of their hearing impaired parent in order to facilitate communication, especially if they are rewarded by the interaction feeling warmer and more complete. When older, some children will feel pleasure from the helpfulness of their actions.

Barbara and Ben encouraged Edward and Louise to perceive their mother's hearing loss as a 'frustration', to be experienced alongside other frustrations of childhood. This raises the question as to whether they were depriving their children of the perspective of seeing their mother as both normal and deaf. Perhaps Barbara and Ben were overprotecting their children and themselves from this enriched perspective because they really didn't know how to manage to communicate it positively. The reality of a disability can be presented to children without undue stress as long as it is accompanied with suitable reassurance. If managed sensitively, it may in fact lead to a new closeness between parents and children and a reduction of the frustration. Counselling can facilitate this process (Grimshaw, 1991; Segal and Simkins, 1993).

Stage III: Families with school children (aged 6–12)

The family is reorganized once again to fit into the expanding world of school children. The family system now overlaps on a regular basis with other systems such as educational, religious and community. Although parents may feel less important once their children start at school and get involved in community activities, child development theory suggests that only a shift of need has taken place. This was illustrated vividly by four latency aged children in the study, Lisa, Louise, Tony and James, who gave explicit messages that they wanted a closer relationship with their parents than they had.

One example was Tony, Anthony's eldest son aged eight. During a private interview with the deafened interviewer, Tony asked:

Is it hard to be deaf?

It was felt that this was a question Tony would have liked to ask his father directly, but was slightly fearful of his response. Tony also recalled:

> and [the] most difficult thing is when [my dad is] in the bedroom and he locks the door. When you want to tell him something, he can't hear.

Barbara's daughter, Louise, aged nine, echoed Tony's complaint. These two eldest children could handle the physical deafness of their parents on its own with equanimity, but it became difficult when compounded with a closed door. While all parents need their privacy from time to time, children often require considerable maturity not to perceive withdrawal behind a closed door, if only temporary, as exclusion. Tony recalled some good experiences:

> sometimes ... [my Dad] gets what we're saying ... the first time he gets close to the word, the second time he gets the word ... or if the second time he doesn't, we help him.

Tony knew he could help his father, but did not appear to feel overly responsible. There seemed to be an understanding amongst the whole family that doing things for Anthony would not reverse the parenting role, as helping was seen in the larger context of satisfying a temporary need within the parent/child relationship. Tony also knew that his hearing mother was there and all the children believed in her capacity to 'make him listen'.

It is significant that Tony used the word 'listen' rather than 'hear' suggesting that he and his siblings were more concerned with their father's capacity for concentration and understanding rather than the biological capacity 'to hear' (Ree, 1999).

Children of the opposite sex from the hearing impaired parent may receive more reassurance in some circumstances. Clare and Anthony's only daughter, Betty, aged six, was allowed to climb up on to her father's lap and test out her power/caring fantasies that she could make him hear by yelling in his ear! In discovering that her efforts were useless, it might at first be disappointing; but she could also be reassured that she was in no way responsible for her father's condition and therefore need feel no guilt about it (Segal and Simkins, 1993).

Conversely, James aged eight at the time his mother was deafened, did not apparently receive this reassurance. This was reflected in James' way of coping which was to simulate a kind of deafness in himself by spending much of his free time in his bedroom when he had formerly been a sociable little boy. Because of their socialization, it is likely that daughters more than sons will be aware of parental vulnerabilities as well as feeling less threatened by them, and therefore, more able to ask for direct reassurance about them.

Children of this age had other ways of coping with their anxiety. For example, Tony worked at getting his facts straight. He recalled:

> My Dad didn't used to be deaf. When I was about two or three, he was all right ... so that's when he became deaf ... because he had this drug in hospital ... he nearly died.'

Being knowledgeable about when his father was deafened in relation to himself appeared reassuring; like his sister, he need not feel responsible. His parents could also recall Tony asking:

> Was it an operation you had on your abdomen?

Being informed about how and where his father was deafened was also an important matter for him. Lastly, being knowledgeable about his father's exact limitations seemed to help. He recalled matter-of-factly:

> and when he's speaking on the phone, ... he can't hear anyone talk. He has to just talk.

All these older children who were able to think in a rational conceptual way identified with their parents and their troubles. Tony, with his parents' support, had done exceptionally well in clarifying what had occurred. The only area he expressed uncertainty about was his father's feelings.

Generally, it could be said that none of the children at this age in the study were subject to inappropriate pressure from an overdependent hearing impaired parent. On occasion this has been known to be a problem and children have been allowed to become too powerful as their parents' 'ears' or as interpreters (Preston, 1994). However this is more likely the case when both parents are deaf. Arthur who had found himself in this situation recalled:

> when I was growing up [I did feel a responsibility to help my parents], ... now I ... [interpret] out of a sense of duty ... everyday things like making appointments with bank managers ... impatient people ... like the Inland Revenue, I have to supervise the whole thing.

Arthur, however, did not feel overburdened by these duties and enjoyed them to a certain extent. There were also no signs that children experienced difficulties in language acquisition. In other words, none of the children had delayed speech development nor had they picked up any signs of deaf speech. The fact that this rarely happens has now been well documented (Schiff-Meyers, 1982).

The children in this study were not, however, as anxiety free about parental deafness as their parents thought. In fact evidence emerged that parents' endeavours to protect their children and themselves by not discussing the hardships of deafness probably led to lost opportunities for interaction and warmer relationships in some families. It was also noticed that the children's behaviour and spirits were in no way oppressed by the formidable quality of parental deafness. This was observed in the way the children were prepared to test limits and make bids for attention in much the same way as children of hearing parents. It is likely that the presence of the parent whose hearing was dependable gave sufficient security to compensate for the extra anxiety the children sometimes felt (Sainsbury, 1986).

There is evidence that children at this age are just beginning to become aware of attitudes of people outside the family, to the disability of deafness generally and their parent's disability specifically (Wolff, 1991). For example, Barbara recalled how her nine-year-old daughter, Louise, reported that another child had asked her why her mother had a 'funny voice'. This had resulted in an uncharacteristically protective response from Louise:

> She's the best mother there is!

Preston (1994) recalls the views of Linda, another child of deaf parents, as she looked back on a childhood which contained similar tensions. Linda recalled:

> Growing up, I was teased a lot. Kids made fun of how Mom talked. They made fun of her expressions. And you know, it was hard to separate it out. But in my house, that's my Mom. That's her way. That's what we do ... (1994: 193)

Both Louise and Linda were struggling with how to sort out family and societal versions of normality.

Stage IV: Families with adolescents

At this stage the family reorganizes to fit into the adolescent's need for a rooted family to which it may return from individuating experiences (Schlesinger, 1986). Marital satisfaction is likely to be at its lowest and stress at its highest. This is because, as families move from the earlier stages of development into adolescence, family cohesiveness decreases resulting in the family's increasing interaction with its environment.

Some researchers suggest that children, teenagers, and daughters of all ages, are particularly impatient with deafened people and sometimes deliberately provoke their hearing impaired parents (Beattie, 1981; Thomas, 1984). Daughters, especially during adolescence, may vacillate between a caring and non-caring role depending upon whether they are feeling closer to a caring mother or a career orientated father (Hare-Mustin, 1978). Other researchers find the opposite pattern in that teenagers are found to be consistently tolerant, cooperative and supportive (Lamont, Harris and Thomas, 1981).

However, Joe's teenage sons had never adjusted to their father's severe hearing difficulties and even denied its existence. Anne's son, Rupert, aged 15, appeared to be more aware of his mother's milder loss. Anne recalled:

> I think Rupert does know [I'm a bit deaf as he] does occasionally get cross. He yelled ... recently when I asked for repetition, 'You are deaf, you are' ... perhaps he was being factual as well as insulting ... it's his way of relating to us.

Anne didn't feel that Rupert was particularly supportive, but then she hadn't raised him to be. His behaviour contrasted sharply with Shirley Ackehurst's (1989) three teenage daughters. They so strongly identified with their deafened mother that each had to have their hearing tested as they reached puberty in an effort to reassure themselves that they could, in fact, hear normally.

There is no explanation given in the literature for why teenagers vary so much other than it being a natural reflection of the range of maturity. Certainly, the model provided by the hearing spouse was an important factor. For example if the hearing partner is calm and patient as in the case of Rachel and Shirley's husbands, their children are likely to follow suit to a certain extent. Conversely, if the hearing parent is impatient as was the case with Sam's wife, the children are likely to emulate this behaviour.

Stage V: Young adult launching

At this stage, the family reorganizes into an egalitarian unit and releases its members. Depending upon the state of the marriage, this may be a time of liberation for the couple, a time of mourning and sadness, or a combination of both. It may also be experienced differently with the wife feeling one way, and the husband feeling another (Bart, 1970). Paradoxically fathers, perhaps realizing they have missed most of the intimacy of their children's development, may begin to seek a closeness from their wives which they have missed; while women after years of focusing on caring for others, begin to feel energized about developing their own lives, careers, and friendships outside the family (McGoldrick, 1991).

American Rachel and English Richard had two sons: William (19) and John (17). Leaving home meant going to the USA either to attend university or to travel. Although in some ways this was a very painful time particularly for Rachel, it was softened by the fact that both boys had chosen to explore her homeland. William and John were proud of being half American and were both interested in working in the film industry in the USA.

Although William and John might inherit their mother's otosclerosis, a conductive hearing loss requiring her to wear two aids, neither son was concerned about this. They knew that their mother had been far more unhappy about other aspects of her life, for example, that she was living in England where she felt she was not fully appreciated, and that she and their father, Richard, were not more compatible. In the past Rachel and Richard, a self-employed accountant, had in fact had a years' marital counselling; but Rachel felt nothing really changed. On numerous occasions in her frustration, she had considered leaving the marriage and returning to the USA. She had not done this as she knew she had become a relative success as a 'Londoner'.

It was understandable that, as her sons left home, Rachel's feelings of loss were reawakened. She used the research interviews to express some of her frustration and to rethink her priorities. Although Rachel and Richard denied any link between her hearing loss and their marital tensions, it was likely that there were subtle connections. Even a very mild hearing loss can prevent a person from displaying the capacity for vivacity, an excellent memory, an alert and powerful integrative intelligence and even humour (Rabbit, 1986). Because Rachel had such a powerful, dramatic personality and was a dedicated university lecturer in the process of completing her doctorate, her hearing loss had not masked any of these qualities in which in fact she excelled.

However, Rachel's personality also resulted in a certain imbalance with her husband and sons. Indeed, they resented the demands her 'highly strung' personality put on their own quieter male natures leaving them largely unsympathetic to her loneliness and isolation. Since members of families often seek reparation for past negative feelings, it is possible that in becoming interested in the film industry in the USA, Rachel's sons were attempting to transform their attitudes.

Stage VI: The middle years: a four generation family

The concept of 'middle age' suggests that on the one hand there is an emphasis on rebirth and fulfilling one's potential; and on the other, there is depression and sadness resulting from unattained goals and being menopausal.

During this stage, reorganization around the marital partner continues as the children are now away most of the time. There is also the possibility of marital satisfaction increasing and continuing into the next stage (Olson and Wilson, 1982).

Frank and Simone, the study couple representative of this stage, were very much in the tradition of the pivotal middle generation. They were effective planners and decision makers and were particularly sensitive to the needs of the generation above and below them (Rapoport, Rapoport, and Strelitz, 1977). They had twins, a boy and a girl, who were now both married with careers and children of their own. Frank and Simone owned a second home in Provence, and it was here that four generations of the family gathered at Easter and Christmas.

Frank eventually acknowledged his mild sensorineural hearing loss in his mid fifties when he was given two NHS hearing aids. He then established a discriminating routine for wearing them as he did not wish for more amplification than absolutely necessary.

While Frank's hearing loss caused him some frustration as it diminished his control and choice in certain circumstances, Simone was not particularly sensitive to this as she tended to compare his condition to her father's more severe loss.

Because of this comparison, Simone's account was that Frank's hearing loss was simply not a problem. While she was aware that the television was now usually on a bit louder, in certain respects, this was just another difference in preference between them. There was the implicit suggestion that learning to cope over time with their basic cultural differences, in being English and French, had prepared them to some extent for all other differences such as hearing loss. On a more intimate and private level, Frank admitted to being 'told off' occasionally by Simone for pretending to hear when he couldn't. Simone reflected on how she saw their relationship at this stage:

> I think we've reached an understanding where we're more willing to talk [things over], and I'm more willing to put my point of view more calmly ... we've grown up.

After a long struggle, they had found a more peaceful civilized way of being that seemed to suit them both for Simone added:

> We [also] have long silences, but they're meaningful.

Frank and Simone knew that some silences were not always meaningful especially with Simone's father. When they were at their holiday home in Provence, they did their best to improve the quality of his life. They also welcomed the youngest members of their family including their three grandsons aged 8, 5 and 3, bringing the total to ten guests. Simone recalled their grandchildren interacting with their great grandfather:

> It was very sweet to watch ... the little ones and my father ... although they didn't speak the same language ... they got on with gestures, and they cuddled ... They watched TV together ...

Dialogue between the very young and the very old appeared to be a less important factor in establishing family rapport than a simple presence and an appreciation of children. Frank remembered how he responded to his father-in-law:

> we were cleaning up the house and [I] had a glass of beer ... and sat down next to [my father-in-law] and talked to him and that was all right. He asked questions and I answered them slowly and ... [we had a chat] ...

Frank also made an effort with his grandsons, He recalled:

> A lot of ... times ... [my grandsons] are simply recounting what they've done and ... seen, ... sometimes ... I find it difficult to follow exactly what it is [they are on about] ... I usually keep it going by saying, 'Mm ... yes ... sure ... mm!' But [they've] got used to me and I say to [them], 'Come a little bit closer if there is something important you want to tell me ...'

Since Frank persisted patiently, he was rewarded in acquiring a certain level of closeness with his grandsons.

The example of Frank and Simone suggests that regardless of hearing impairment, the so called 'empty nest' period can be a time of great range and involvement, when the marital partners are more secure and at peace with each other, with their careers and the wider community, and with their parents, grown-up children, and grandchildren.

Obviously all families are not as fortunate as this. Illnesses can occur and mental health deteriorate. In this small study alone, one couple divorced, and one hearing impaired husband had a massive heart attack and died.

It emerged that cross generational misunderstandings about hearing impairment were more likely to occur in step families. An example of this occurred when Sarah's two grandsons came to visit some years after she married her second husband, Joe. She recalled the following incident:

> So we are in the kitchen ... [My grandsons] came in with their toys on the floor ... just to be near us ... but you see they want to talk to each other, and I'm wanting to tell Joe about something that happened to me at work last week ... and the boys keep talking, and Joe was getting cross ...

Eventually with so much tension about, Joe's patience snapped and he became angry at one of his step grandsons. It was at some cost to Sarah for she continued:

> and I was so hurt ... for Joe because he hadn't understood what ... [the little boy had] said, and just as hurt for the little boys. They were trying their best to understand and I'd had ... to stand them together and say, 'You know, Granddad can not hear a thing without his hearing aid ... but his hearing aid makes everything too loud, but ... a little five year old and seven year old can't understand that, and it's pretty awful.

Sarah was a proficient mediator, although not without considerable 'role strain'. Joe was not unsympathetic to his grandsons' viewpoints for he added:

> I walked out of the room ... I didn't want to make the situation worse than it was ... I was quite upset too ... not for myself, but for the children because it's frustrating.

Peace was eventually restored. Sarah recalled:

> In the afternoon, Joe was sitting over there and my other grandson said to him, 'Can I come and have a cuddle, Granddad?' ... and he just went and sat on his lap ... and I said, 'Granddad loves you. He'll always be here to look after you ... you both know that' ... but it was an uncomfortable half an hour ...

While step parenting may be delicate when one partner has a hearing loss, as we have seen, natural grandparents also have their difficulties. It is possible that the more recent bonding of step parents will make competition and insecurity a stronger feature of intimate relationships with children (Burgoyne and Clark, 1984).

Stage VII: Retirement and ageing (male over 65)

The emergence of retirement is one of the most significant social trends of the past fifty years (Phillipson, 1987). It is the stage in the life-cycle when hearing loss becomes a common condition usually in the form of presbycusis. This was the diagnosis of four people in the study: Robert, Theo, Max and Frank.

Robert (70) had also contracted Menière's Disease just prior to his retirement. Besides losing his hearing within a period of six months, he also experienced attacks of vertigo, blinding headaches and tinnitus. Robert confronted his illness head on by taking sign language and lip reading courses. Eventually, he discovered the radio microphone as an assisting device and used it on a regular basis with family, friends, and in the community groups he attended and chaired.

Although grown-up children are not as vulnerable as younger ones, Robert's adult children, nevertheless, were deeply affected by his condition. By interviewing three of his four children, along with his wife Mary, a rounded picture of the most pronounced attitude changes emerged.

Robert's eldest son, David, a psychologist, put the family's initial reaction in context by explaining how his father had formerly been a passive, but responsible parent. It was their mother, Mary, who was the important one. Occasionally, Robert would emerge from behind his books and ask for repetition of bits of family conversation. David recalled:

> I think [Dad] wanted to be in control of what he had access to ... so in a sense everything you said had to be available to him, but the choice was his ...

David's observations support the literature and the generally understood role of the husband/father as controller of information (Kyle, Jones and Wood, 1985). However, there was a second level of meta-communication that was taking place within this family (Tannen, 1986). David added:

> the deafness took away his choice in the matter ... we would make some very silly comment ... we would have to repeat it three times ... we could never get away with saying the standard thing 'it doesn't matter' because it always did ...

Robert, like Max (see Chapter 8), knew implicitly that so called 'trivial' conversations were important in that they reinforced a feeling of 'belonging' in some families. However, Robert did not know how to articulate his needs appropriately. David recalled:

> There were occasions when ... [Dad] was very hurt [and there was a lot of anger around], ... there certainly was an element of 'if you cared for me, you'd [include me in your discussions]' ... maybe I reacted like it was a manipulation ... [which] may have been ... unjust to him.

At this point Robert's hearing loss became a 'stressor' as the family did not have the resources to effectively handle it (Oyer and Oyer, 1985). David continued:

> We are an articulate family up to a point, but there ... [are] quite a lot of things we would not talk about, and I think the question of people's feelings comes below the line ... I think it's a habit rather than an actual taboo ...

An unpredictable family crisis had occurred. This meant the family's intellectual culture which did not discuss feelings (Handel, 1985) initially lacked the resources to manage Robert's deafness without precipitating further anger and stress (Joselevich, 1988). Because Robert was unable to articulate directly how frustrated he felt, the development of his children's compassionate feelings for him was delayed.

Robert's hearing loss has been considered in terms of how it affected his family as a group. Changes also occurred individually with each child. For example, David acknowledged how his father's deafness caused them to become more supportive of each other and less competitive as they faced together Robert's genuine limitations. David recalled:

> people might say ... Dad's more at ease with [his disability than he was], ... I think you see that more in [our debates], ... he and I are happier to agree to disagree than we were three or four years ago.

Thus, for David, their debating passion had dissipated into some sort of acceptance of the situation. Robert's relationship with his younger son, Paul, also changed. He had always admired his father greatly, but felt it impossible to keep up with him intellectually. Eventually Paul found work in the post office as a telegraphist. Later he was transferred to Brussels and worked for the European Economic Commission operating a telex machine. Sadly, his emotional health deteriorated. Eventually he had a nervous breakdown not long after his father was diagnosed as having Menière's Disease. As Robert was now retired, he went to live with Paul in Brussels for three years attempting to help him regain his mental health and competence. Unfortunately, Paul's health remained unstable, and eventually they both returned to England. Initially, Paul recalled being upset by his father's deafness since it made Robert fall off the 'parental pedestal' he had made for him. It had taken ten years for Paul and Robert to rebuild their relationship, this time based on mutual acceptance and a deeper understanding of their own and each others' humanity. Paul reflected:

> I think we get on better if we go to a restaurant and we are face to face ... then [my Dad] can see my facial movements, lips, teeth, eyes, and I can see him and then realize, 'Oh that is my dad' you know.

Although Paul was still officially 'mentally ill' in that he was periodically readmitted to a psychiatric day hospital for treatment, he was, nevertheless, poignantly sensitive to the way his relationship with his father had become more reciprocal in certain situations.

Robert's role in his younger daughter's life had also been crucial. Molly, a mother and GP, sensed early on how frustrated her father was professionally. Perhaps because Robert had not found job fulfilment on lower levels, he had encouraged all his children to reach for the top regardless of gender or disability. Molly was pleased to see how her father was able to practise what he preached by gaining back his old confidence with family and strangers. She recalled one incident the previous Christmas:

> My husband had just written a Pantomime ... for the family, and my father was one of the Ugly Sisters and ... [Dad] had the rather unkind name of 'deaf-as-a-Post Purveyor', but he didn't mind ... he had his words and one of the grandchildren would just prod him when it was time to speak, ... he was wonderful.

Adjustments were also required for Robert's wife, Mary. David and Molly knew how Robert's disability often left Mary feeling quite isolated. Molly said:

> I'm aware how lonely it has been for ... [Mum]. She loves to ... be in a conversation, ... she doesn't like silence. If she can't think of anything to say, she'll sing ... so I think [Dad's deafness] has been very hard for her and I am aware that she has been low over the past few years ...

Mary was likely to be mourning a certain loss of domestic sociability as Sarah in Chapter 5 described. Mary recalled:

> when I see other couples together ... chatting, ... you do realize you're missing out ... [as Robert] always used to be joking and quoting poetry and singing ... occasionally we get sparks of it now ... I suppose it is the hearing problem a lot of it. Maybe I don't respond the right way ... we change, don't we?

Mary and Robert's spirits were undoubtedly dampened by all the 'unpredictable crises' in the family which occurred in a relatively short period (1979–85). However, such a 'pile up' of stressful events is not unusual in family life (Walsh, 1998). Nevertheless, the need for practical strategies to manage Robert's specific deafness remained. He explained:

> Our ... children ... will forget ... They start talking together and I just cannot follow what they're saying ... So there I am standing in a group ... but not of the group ... Maybe they don't want me to ... [be there]. If I could hear what they're saying, I'd know whether I was part of the conversation or not ... so there is difficulty, although ... on the whole, they're pretty good.

Robert's relationships with his grandchildren varied. In some ways he found it easier to relate to his Canadian grandchildren since they played badminton, tennis and computer games with him. It was also probable that as products of North American culture, they were less fearful than their English counterparts of speaking up to adults.

Regardless of Robert and David's breakdown in health, Robert and Mary were helped to mobilize their natural resiliency (Walsh, 1998) by receiving excellent medical and psychological guidance. Their level of functioning and feelings of well-being gradually improved, making it possible for them to continue with community commitments as well as family ones, although Robert often needed Mary's support in his endeavours.

Summary

The literature in the field of acquired hearing loss has oversimplified the discussion of the impact of acquired hearing impairment on children's lives and so this chapter has focused primarily on the study of children's attitudes and feelings, and an effort has been made to analyse their responses to acquired hearing loss in one of their parents.

There were a number of factors which persisted throughout the whole life-cycle. It appeared to be the case that deafness could have a negative impact on children in that it made them worry or feel resentful, but that these feelings could be modified by sensitive management of the disability and the children.

Although the children in the study were encouraged to facilitate lip-reading by facing their hearing impaired parent when speaking, suggesting some control, none of them seemed to feel the sort of awesome responsibility which can occur when both parents are deaf. There appeared to be a direct connection between their relatively relaxed attitude and the fact that the hearing parent was present and had a stable relationship with their hearing impaired parent. There was a tremendous range found in 'when' parents told 'what' to their children about deafness. Some parents started as early as three or four years of age with articulated explanations in response to their child(ren)'s growing awareness that something was slightly different about Mummy or Daddy, while others preferred a more laid-back 'wait and see' approach. The first approach was supported by parents who wished to instil a strong sense of responsibility in their children, while the second approach was initiated by parents who wished to preserve their children's innocence as long as possible. It is argued that the latter approach may protect children and their parents from the enriched perspective of understanding the hearing impaired parent as being both deaf and normal, different and the same.

There was no support for the view that children, specifically adolescents, may reject their hearing impaired parent and that grandchildren inevitably upset their hearing impaired grandparents. On the contrary, it was found that grandchildren, like children, will make appropriate adjustments if helped to do so. When grandparents experienced difficulty, they were usually those who had not had positive experiences with children in the past or did not particularly like children.

Thus, the evidence reinforces the idea that rehabilitators of hearing impaired people need to have a sound grasp of the family life-cycle approach and to have some understanding of the 'role strains' which are experienced.

From an examination of family life, the focus moves to the development of kin and friendship networks when one partner is hearing impaired.

CHAPTER 8

Kinship networks

Introduction

The importance of social networks cannot be overestimated. Researchers have even suggested that the natural immune system is to the body as the kin-friendship network is to the individual (Broderick, 1988).

Although research has begun into the social networks of so called deprived and disabled groups, there is little in the literature pertaining to the networks of people with acquired hearing loss. This is not a reflection of the perceived lack of importance of social networks for hearing impaired people. On the contrary, this study supports the literature when it suggests that the degree of psychological distress experienced by people with a hearing loss is more closely correlated to the level of social support given from social networks than to the actual degree of impairment (Frankel and Turner, 1983).

However, it emerged in this study that hearing impaired people do not receive the support of sufficient quality from their kin that is conventionally assumed, a problem which is partly culturally based. By culture is meant 'highly specific systems that both explain things and constrain how things can be known' (Padden and Humphries, 1988: 24).

The three levels of social network formation suggested by Unger and Powell (1980) are used here in order to provide a context within which the experiences of the people interviewed in the present study may be understood.

Social networks: general definition and characteristics

Social networks may be defined as a collection of individuals who know and interact with a particular target individual or couple (Fischer, 1982; Milardo, 1988). The interactions are the specific exchanges which take place between people; they occur in the present moment.

The literature suggests that the value of the term 'network' lies in avoiding the reification connected in talking about 'community', yet enabling one to talk about a wider set of informal relationships than just the family or the extended kin group. The set of relationships is broadened to include friends, neighbours and work associates (Bulmer, 1987).

Some individuals are more socially active than others, for example extroverts more than introverts, which results in size variations of social networks. Other factors which could contribute to size variations are level of education, occupation, income, physical attributes such as attractiveness (Reis *et al.*, 1982), relatively stable personal disposition (Perlman, 1988), social skills (Burns and Farina, 1984), location, and the stage in the life-cycle (Dickens and Perlman, 1981).

The formation of traditional social networks

Class (Willmott, 1986), gender (Allan, 1989) and ethnicity (Willmott, 1986) have emerged in the last two decades as the three most traditional factors to influence social network formation. More recently additional factors have been examined specifically in relation to more deprived groups. For example, there are studies of the social networks of elderly people (Adams, 1986), disabled people (Schilling, Gilchrist and Schinke, 1984) and injured pensioners (Sainsbury, 1993). Lastly, there are studies of the social networks of people progressing through expected and unexpected life change or crisis, such as transitions to motherhood, divorce, and transitions through the life-cycle more generally (O'Brien, 1985).

Although the literature discusses the social networks of the profoundly deaf who are members of the Deaf culture (Padden and Humphries, 1988; Harris, 1995), there is very little on the social networks of people with acquired hearing impairment. It is, in fact, there, but absorbed in general studies of people with disabilities (Townsend, 1963).

Perhaps the paucity of literature on this topic reflects a number of factors. First, the needs of people with acquired hearing impairment are often confused with people who are prelingually deaf and are part of the Deaf culture. Consequently the needs of people with acquired hearing loss have only recently emerged. Secondly, because acquired hearing loss suggests a breakdown in communication, this in turn suggests the incapacity of people with this disability to initiate and sustain a credible social network. Unlike prelingually deaf people, there is no culture, language, or 'reference group' to fall back on (Hyman, 1942). Thirdly, the concept of 'social network' itself is relatively new in the literature.

The composition of traditional social networks

Traditionally social networks are made up of a certain balance of kin, neighbours and friendships. This also holds true for the social networks of the hearing impaired. It is helpful to differentiate these three terms before considering the case of hearing impaired people.

Kin relations are long-term ties whether or not there is regular face-to-face contact. Ties with neighbours are face-to-face contacts and often time-dependent as with borrowing small necessities or help in emergencies. Ties with friends have an affective basis reinforced by common interests or experience, and may or may not involve frequent face-to-face contacts.

Given these different functions, as sources of care, kin, friends and neighbours tend to complement each other in meeting different types of need at different times, rather than being substitutes for one another. However, it is argued that some substitution does take place in the creativeness of everyday life, particularly in providing psychological support and domestic care.

In the final analysis, it is suggested that kinship ties are qualitatively different from those with friends and neighbours. Although too much emphasis may be placed on the obligatory character of kinship, it remains true that as a source of long-term commitment, kinship ties are pre-eminent. In all major crises, it is to kin people first turn. However, paradoxically, kin support in practice has an unpredictable quality about it and the following factors need to be considered as indicators of who gives what to whom: gender, ethnicity, generation and economic position (Willmott, 1986; Bott, 1957).

Gender also represents a principle through which different treatment is filtered. For example male and female relations are treated differently in many cases even when they both fall into the inner circle.

Until recently, the only evidence regarding networks of people with hearing impairment has come from studies which focus more broadly on disability. It is to these that we now turn to consider how the experience of disability affects the general picture of kinship networks.

Social support networks when there is disability in the family: three social support levels

Support networks for families where there is disability appear to require more structure because of the extra stress and vulnerability experienced (Voysey, 1975; Rapoport, Rapoport and Strelitz, 1977). Unger and Powell (1980) have identified three levels of social support when there is a disability in the family. First, there is the nuclear family, close friends and relatives, and other significant persons. A second level of support includes neighbours, more distant friends and relatives, and certain professional and service providers. Although less intimate than the first level of support, these sources of help typically have regular contact with the family. A third level of support is still less intimate and is defined by superficial or infrequent contact often in the context of social institutions. The ability to interact skilfully with others rather than circumstances alone is believed to be the most important factor when building a social network (Gottlieb, 1981). The success of families seeking social support, in whatever form, will to a large extent depend on their social competence (for example, in articulation of need, arranging reciprocal exchanges, and in responding appropriately when the needs of others change).

However, the tasks of network building cannot entirely lie on the shoulders of disabled people and their families who are likely to be (but not always) in a disadvantaged position to handle them. Some of the specific barriers to social network formation experienced by the hearing impaired will be outlined now.

Barriers to network formation when there is hearing impairment in the family

People with acquired hearing impairment are likely to experience more difficulty than hearing people in forming social networks since the disability itself strikes at communication, the heart of social discourse. Loneliness specifically caused by deafness appears to contain two distinct components; 'social isolation' (that is the result of an apparent inability to sustain and maintain a social network in the outside world), and 'emotional isolation' (that is the inability to be involved and understood by one's immediate family) (Thomas and Herbst, 1980).

Sloss Luey (1980) focuses on the intensity of the deafened person's feelings which may threaten or repel potential friends especially when they are excluded from the easy sociability which depends on not only the meaning, but also the context and inflection of words, quick repartee, interruptions, jokes, nuances and word play. On the other hand, research suggests old friends are lost and new friends made during any major life transition (Askham, 1984).

Despite various barriers to creating social networks, the findings of this study suggest that they may be overcome to a certain extent as we will now see.

Kinship support in the social networks of hearing impaired people

In general some kinship support could be counted upon by hearing impaired people. However, there was considerable variation in the kind and quality of support given.

Kinship support in culturally mixed marriages

The most comprehensive support was provided by Beatrice and Andrew, parents of Gwen. She and her Deaf husband, Arthur, formed the 'newly wed couple' in this study. Beatrice and Andrew had previous experience with disability in that their elder daughter, Rebecca, had contracted an arthritic condition not long after she married.

While Beatrice acknowledged that she and Andrew had not wished to endorse all the traditions from their home, the Isle of Lewis; that of 'hospitality' was one to which they both aspired. Beatrice explained how it was that Arthur's parents, Sue and Rob, spent Christmas week with them for the second year in succession:

> Christmas of last year was the first Christmas after [Gwen and Arthur] were married ... I said, 'I can manage to give everybody lunch,' and (my other daughter), Rebecca said ' ... I'll do the supper' ... and that is what we did ...

Perhaps mixed with the hospitality tradition was an altruistic ideal that people should help people who need help (Gouldner, 1960). Also having a joint family Christmas appeared the best way of resolving fantasies, competitive feelings, and doubts particularly when an 'outsider' (Higgens, 1980) is married to an 'insider', or from a cultural perspective, marriage occurs 'across frontiers' (Barbara, 1989).

However, Beatrice and Andrew were wise enough to be aware that the giving went both ways and felt it to be a privilege to help Arthur. They were keenly aware of Arthur's need to achieve a level appropriate to his formidable intellect and literary ability.

Although Beatrice and Andrew willingly gave their encouragement, strict boundaries were observed to avoid the danger of over involvement or enmeshment (Harvey, 1989). Beatrice related:

> The choice(s) must be ... [theirs, and] Arthur likes to talk to Andrew about [things] ... he'll consult him on the wording of a letter, ... since Andrew has been through the university system ... as well as Gwen, Rebecca and Geoff ...

'Enmeshment' or its opposite 'disengagement' (Galvin and Brommel, 1991) are often psychological threats to families where there is a disability. It may be asked how this couple managed to keep such a clear sense of appropriate boundaries. Beatrice pointed to her friendship circle as being helpful:

> We've always been fortunate in our own friends; and so we have a wonderful circle of friends ...

Discussions with close friends helped Beatrice and Andrew maintain their objectivity, equilibrium, and sense of mastery or control when faced with family disability (Kazak and Marvin, 1984). Gwen, however, appeared only aware of her parents' acceptance and identified with it. She related:

> [Perhaps] ... the way ... [my parents] brought me up has meant that they can cope, and I can cope with ... [Arthur] [and] his deafness ...

Gwen reflected a sensitivity to what Krebs (1970) calls 'a subterranean nexus of reciprocity'. Because her parents were caring compassionate people, she was also. She went on to describe her parents' initiative in attempting to learn BSL:

> My father's ... shy so he's ... wary of using Sign, but he will finger spell if he's ... [repeated without Arthur understanding] ... My Mum signs a bit more ... [as] she's an extrovert.

While Gwen implied that personality is one factor in willingness to use and learn BSL, the primary issue is seen as one of acceptance. For both Gwen and Arthur, this gesture was symbolic of her parents' acceptance (Harris, 1995) of Arthur and Deaf people generally (Higgens, 1980).

Andrew and Beatrice's BSL initiative could also be seen as a symbol of 'intergenerational solidarity' (Bengston and Cutler, 1976). Three key factors composed the solidarity that existed between Andrew, Beatrice and Arthur. The first factor is 'association'. The more Beatrice and Andrew associated with Arthur, the more solidarity existed within the relationship. Within the literature, association has been typically defined as close interpersonal contact and residential propinquity. A second factor is 'affection'. Bengston and his colleagues argue that helping behaviour is the key signal to affection within a relationship and the giving of help is the crucial element. The third factor related to family solidarity is a certain mutuality of values, beliefs and opinions. Any behaviour that aided this 'consensus' promoted solidarity. Since Andrew, Beatrice and Arthur had similar values regarding education, religion and equal opportunities, a common value base truly existed.

Although Arthur acknowledged that he had never felt so much acceptance, communication was difficult with Andrew. Arthur recalled:

> when ... my father-in-law Signs, he is very stiff ... [and] he keeps Signing to a bare minimum ... I think he feels more comfortable with finger spelling ... he's [also] very difficult to lip-read ... because he's got a very strong Scottish accent.

Gwen too recounted communication problems, but more with her mother:

> Mum found it very difficult at first ... if we were talking [in Sign] and I'd switched off my voice. She would forget that we were talking ... She would talk to me and then she'd be upset because I didn't answer because I was talking [using Sign with Arthur] ...

Gwen's sensitivity to linguistic exclusion was understandable as she had found it difficult as a child to hear her parents speak their native Gaelic, a language she was never taught. While visiting Beatrice and Andrew during the Christmas holidays, Arthur's Deaf parents made the following remarks about living with a hearing family:

Rob:

> it's hard, ... you don't know what [the family] are saying.

Sue:

> Sometimes Gwen talks [without Signing] to her parents, but it doesn't worry me. Sometimes Gwen tells me what it is.

At this time Arthur's parents were also Gwen and Arthur's neighbours. Such close proximity could make the relationship a powerful instrument for informal care as illustrated in studies of working-class families (Young and Willmott, 1972; Cornwell, 1984). However, unless an element of 'choice' was experienced, there was danger that the relationship would deteriorate into one of obligation and enmeshment.

Arthur felt his parents, specifically his father, had been socialized into feelings of dependence and powerlessness and that his father perceived himself as not having the cognitive competence, psychological skills and support systems needed to influence his environment successfully (Schlesinger, 1985).

Barbara and Ben provided another example of intergenerational solidarity as they had worked hard from the beginning to consciously eradicate any condescension in her husband's family. Barbara felt her best advocate was her own attitude. She explained:

> Often in [my] marriage [my] positiveness makes it fairly easy for my relatives to accept me. [For them], I am probably a force to be reckoned with, ... well I am not a 'poor little thing' ... there are difficult situations such as large family gatherings ... and I don't hear everything that is said, but that happens everywhere.

Barbara was reluctant to make traditional English assumptions concerning the reliability of female kin support (Finch, 1989). This was not because of a lack of trust, but rather that 'the care' provided would stifle her ambition and drive, personal characteristics which she valued above all others as they had been carefully fostered by her Australian parents.

Although Barbara did not present kin as useful for social support, she did value their companionship on holidays. Unlike Arthur and Gwen's 'at home' family holidays, these were abroad. Barbara recalled:

> we went to Brittany for two weeks ... beautiful weather. My sister and her four children, my mother, my father-in-law ... it was a big family party ... lovely.

Barbara first presented her holiday as a rosy success. Later she revealed that there had been difficulties in which she played a major part to resolve. She remembered:

> My deafness on holiday was an advantage. [Two] car[s] broke down so I volunteered ... to look for a garage ... [There] they were all set for me to phone for ... [one] in French! So I said, 'I'm terribly sorry, I am deaf and cannot use the phone ... would you be very kind and make the telephone call?' ... [which they eventually did] ...

Kinship support also emerged as a factor for elderly people, specifically Max and Theo, a widower and a widow (see Chapter 10). Max's story will begin to unfold in the next section.

Kinship support for elderly hearing impaired people

Before discussing Max, some new understandings of the lives of elderly people will be reviewed. First, the literature suggests that elderly people are not as lonely a group as sometimes supposed. It is probably true that the amount of social contact declines with age (Larson, Zuzanek and Mannell, 1985), but actual levels of contact are not considered to be the crucial factor. Rather it is more important to consider the gap between achieved and desired levels of contact. It may be that the desired level of contact with other people drops as rapidly as actual levels of contact, thus protecting older adults from loneliness. The other factor which emerged is that the contacts which elderly people do have are usually of a higher quality than when younger thus providing more satisfaction.

However, Clark and Anderson (1980) believe that the most critical factors regarding loneliness and elderly people are whether or not they have a confidante and good peer relationships.

Contact with kin is another factor attributed to keeping loneliness at bay for elderly people. Arling (1976), in his study of American widows found that lower levels of loneliness are not related to visits from children, but are related to greater contact with friends and neighbours. While contact with family members may persist, there is no guarantee that it is enjoyable. Rosnow (1967) argues that frequent contact between elderly people and their children often becomes ritualistic, based on obligation rather than warmth or closeness. However, it could also be argued that feelings in more fixed societies than the USA are even more deeply held behind seemingly ritual and conventional behaviour.

Bearing this in mind, it was not surprising to find Max, a distinguished educational administrator with no previous history of hearing loss, fighting to hold on to the remnants of control and independence. Now in his early eighties, he found himself retired, widowed, moderately hearing impaired and isolated to a certain extent.

As with the example of Arthur and Gwen and Gwen's parents, 'care' took the form of respectful concern. In this case, however, the informal care managers were Max's two daughters, Margaret a social worker and Esther a teacher.

A combination of accident and design meant that Margaret and her family lived a few houses down the street from Max making her a neighbour as well as kin. There were, thus, more opportunities for care exchanged between them to be informal, reciprocal, and sometimes enjoyable. This state of affairs was strongly endorsed by Max who needed to be continually reassured that he was not a burden

(Barry, 1995). Nevertheless, there were certain difficulties with communication. Margaret gave an example:

> At the table [my father] will sometimes say, 'Are you speaking to me?' And I say, 'No, not at the moment'. And I feel bad about it because I feel he's not included ... even in the circle of five of us eating together ... unless we speak directly to him ...

It is well documented that 'the dinner table', the symbol of family togetherness and the primary forum for the socialization of children among middle class families, may become a symbol of isolation and even alienation for many hearing impaired individuals (Becker, 1980). Max's family was certainly aware of the problem as Margaret's husband, Colin, recounted:

> [Max] ... likes to know what's going on like most of us do ... he feels excluded because you're not always conscious of his deafness, ... because when [we're] having a conversation, we tend to ... drop our voices ... and we talk about something that has happened between the two of us, which really isn't for his ears anyway ... [maybe something quite trivial] ... but then he says, 'what's happening? ... [or] 'Am I missing out on something?'

Although Max's family did amazingly well in caring for him on a practical level and to some extent on an emotional one as we shall see, these examples highlighted the problematic paradoxical heart of the matter with many English families and their elderly hearing impaired relations. Max knew implicitly that English middle-class domestic norms dictate, by way of their conversational style (Tannen, 1986, 1989), that feelings of 'belonging' are generated by unstated meanings and being privy to the mundane details of everyday domestic life. When a hearing loss prevented their absorption, the situation became more complex because of the traditional English dislike of 'repeating' unless a subject is really important. To this is added the fact that there are enormous ambiguities involved in sensory impairments generally making it difficult for caring relatives to respond appropriately. For example, how does one know whether or not a hearing impaired relation has heard something? Conversely, there is no ambiguity when an elderly relative is in a wheel chair as everyone knows it requires pushing.

It was for these reasons that the hearing impaired people in this study were not closer to their kin. In the next section, illustrations are given where kin were overtly hurtful in that they had left the hearing impaired person feeling fearful and inadequate rather than supported.

When kinship becomes unhelpful, hurtful and/or condescending

It became evident that ambiguities involved in a hearing handicap may in fact result in mistreatment by kin. For example, Joe (aged 64) who had been partially deafened at the age of two by diphtheria reported the following incidents:

> [When] ... I ... [was] ... a child [of] eleven, ... My mother had a cousin of about 19 ... [who] used to tease me ... [as] I couldn't pronounce my 's's' ... I used to say 'Yeah' [instead of Yes]. But a child of that age feels ... [hurt by such criticism]. Then my mother had another cousin. We were a group in a family ... and I started to say something, and they were listening to me and I was talking with my hands ... And [this cousin] said, 'stop talking with your hands. Put your hands under your thighs', which I did and I stopped talking, ... [and ever since] I've always worried that [I was] going to make a fool of myself in company ...

Indeed, some of Joe's first attempts to form his own social network were blocked by insensitive older relations. Joe also had difficulty with his parents whom he felt never really understood his communication needs, nor were they able to help him articulate them to others.

A somewhat similar story was told by Henry. He recalled his relief when both his children were pronounced free from hearing loss:

> it was part of [my social] conditioning ... a lot of it was my relations thinking I was not [a good marriage prospect] ... because of my deafness, ... and some of them had the ... idea that the handicap might be hereditary ... [It deeply affected me and is connected with the fact that I did not marry] until my late thirties ... I know that when Clive was tested in our house in Norfolk, I felt a great sense of relief that everything was all right.

These two examples illustrate the enormous importance of an accepting kinship network for hearing impaired young people when they begin to reach out to make their own circle of friends. Because of these early humiliations at the hands of relations, both

Joe and Henry had to struggle with what is called 'the invalid mind', which develops when people who have been disabled early in life are treated as inferior and consequently develop deep feelings of inferiority.

Yet because condescending attitudes are so prevalent, changing them is of necessity a difficult long-term process. Barbara calls this process 'converting the environment' (1989).

However, the passing of time didn't always make a difference; for example, Julia's parents stubbornly opposed her commitment to Sam. Although she loved all her family, she was proud that she and Sam had kept their independence from them.

Kinship support when there are geographical distance barriers

Two deafened people in the study had migrated from other countries, Nigeria and the United States, so that the distance factor was in fact very great. Both people, a man and a woman, had extroverted personalities and were in high status professions which undoubtedly affected their attitudes and determination to keep in touch with their roots. They seemed to see the distance between England, their resident country, and their country of origin as a challenge rather than an obstacle. Although maintaining contact was hard at times, both had succeeded in doing this through telephone calls, letters, and visits. It was of interest that the network of the Nigerian, Anthony, was dominated by kin while the network of the American, Rachel, was dominated by friends. They also both succeeded in actively building networks in the UK.

Anthony had not only kept his network, he had also sustained his high status within his family (Fortes, 1969). He explained:

> Before decisions are taken in Nigeria on major issues, my family must consult me in writing and wait for my reply. They [have] followed whatever I say up until now ... the realization of my responsibilities as someone interested in my family makes me struggle harder.

Anthony was the eldest of five brothers and sisters. Although he remembered his family as expressing great sorrow when they were told of his deafness, they nevertheless remained loyal. This suggests that in a fairly fixed society such as Nigeria, if a person has a high profile role within their family when they are disabled (deafened), they will keep this status provided they are perceived as carrying on their family duties and responsibilities.

When reviewing the two families discussed most often in this chapter, it was the mothers, Beatrice and Margaret, who were most dedicated in their attempts to care. Fathers had more of a 'watch dog' role, making sure their wives didn't over do it and thus endanger the equilibrium of the rest of the family. The roles played by mothers and fathers will be explored more fully in the next section.

Close kinship support with reference to gender

Gender has been called a prism through which all of our lives are lived. It is ever-present and yet taken for granted. It affects the language we use (Tannen, 1991), the way we move, and our conception of relationships (Gilligan, 1982).Women generally are more involved than men in social support. This is thought to be a matter of necessity rather than choice based upon the division of labour in our society. While both men and women may now go out to work, women on the whole have retained domestic and caring responsibilities for which they need the support of others (Finch, 1989).

Mothers and fathers

The literature suggests that some women devote much of their lives to kinship support (Lewis and Meredith, 1988). Besides the mothers already mentioned, there were two others who might be called 'rehabilitation mothers'. They were women who had experienced tragedy themselves, had survived it, and therefore knew how to bring others through similar experiences of traumatic loss. Sam recalled how his mother responded when he was deafened at aged 17:

> she put up with me ... I suppose to begin with I was very moody and she was very patient and very supportive ... she made me get on with my life. She did not let me stay in bed all day.

Sam's father had been there, but was less helpful because of an ingrained attitude of pessimism. Sam eventually recovered his equilibrium and

went on to become the first member of his family to complete under-
graduate and post graduate education. Perhaps partly because of his
mother's support at the critical time, Sam was prevented from developing the 'invalid mind' (Thunem, 1966) which sometimes occurs. Other
people in the study were less fortunate. Joy recalled her mother's
response at the time when she and Mike had to temporarily move back
into the parental home after she was deafened by meningitis:

> I never really got on with my mother ... and she didn't really take to my deafness
> ... She was quite friendly in her way, ... but she would ignore me every now and
> then ... [and] she turned to my sister ... and I felt a bit left out ... whether it was
> me or my deafness [is not clear].

Although Joy was unlucky with her mother, she was extremely
fortunate in her husband, Mike, who managed her recovery in a not
too dissimilar way as Sam's mother had done for him.

The above examples demonstrate a certain unpredictability
surrounding kinship support. Finch suggests that kinship support is
rarely possible to predict simply from knowing that one has a
mother, a brother, or grandchildren, or what assistance, if any, is to
be given at present or in the future (1989). Assistance is often given,
but how much, from whom, and of what quality can not be assumed.

Siblings

Sibling relationships are similar to that of parents and children in that
both are ascribed (Downing, 1990). They are perceived as different from
these relationships in two important ways. First, although support does
pass between siblings, it seems less reliable, in the sense that whether it is
offered often depends on personal circumstances and personal liking.
Secondly, sibling relationships tend to be much more obviously built
upon reciprocal exchange between two people who are in equivalent
genealogical positions. In both respects the relationships bore a closer
resemblance to voluntary friendship than to kinship (McGhee, 1985).

Rivalry and competition are major functions of sibling relationships in adolescence (Sutton-Smith and Rosenburg, 1970) as they are
thought to be helpful in preparing for later competition and to build
character. Allan (1979) did not find any evidence that sibling rivalry
continued through the life span, although it could arise on occasion.

Both sisters and brothers were mentioned as being helpful by hearing impaired people in this study. Moderately deafened Martha (55), a member of a large Irish family, described how one sister helped:

> I can understand my sister on the telephone because she knows ... I'm deaf and she speaks up ... you see I haven't got confidence in anybody [else] ... only my own people ...

Martha drew a strong social boundary around her female kin calling them implicitly 'special' (Finch, 1989), as they were the only ones she could 'hear' on the telephone.

But siblings also had the power to hurt. Frank, a geography professor in his sixties, related the following incident:

> [my sister] occasionally has ... [referred to my] deafness ... [at a dinner party] ... [She will say], 'Oh,.. [my brother's] deaf you know'. At that moment, it hurts, but then I forget it ...

Frank's wife, Simone, put his sister's tactlessness down to latent sibling rivalry (Sutton-Smith and Rosenberg, 1970). She said:

> I think there has always been a sort of jealousy [that Frank's sister is] not conscious of. Frank has always been his mother's favourite ... and he was the one who academically succeeded and she didn't ...

While there were feelings of rivalry between some siblings, the relationship between Joe and his sister was quite different. Joe's wife, Sarah, told this story as Joe was too moved to tell it:

> Joe's ... sister is in a psychiatric unit ... She tried to come out this year, but ... couldn't cope. I went to see her to help her talk about how she couldn't cope ... it was a classic case of someone who'd been institutionalized ...

This was the most extreme example of the complete breakdown in what might have been a supportive relationship between sister and brother. Where both siblings were hearing impaired, the relationship was more complex. Theo (84) recalled what car outings were like with her much younger sister:

> We went up to Derbyshire ... but I realized that I must not talk ... I can't say 'Oh, look at this, look at that' ... because then she turns around to see ... [and we'd] be in a ditch ...

Although Theo was ambivalent, her relationship with her sister was an active one with many reciprocal aspects. Sarah mentioned how her brother's attitude changed towards Joe's deafness:

> When ... [my brother] first met Joe, he understood about the difficulty, but ... he didn't empathize at all because he was [physically] ok. Then he became diabetic and his whole attitude has changed ...

Thus, Sarah's brother's illness helped him to become sensitized to Joe's need for repetition. Barbara's brother was also helpful as husband Ben explained:

> Barbara's brother is very good at ... [interpreting the television], but he has had many years of practice at it, ... [as] it is really quite difficult to listen to something and tell somebody else about it ...

Barbara's brother is the only example of a male interpreter, a role usually taken by women whether relatives or friends (Preston, 1994). It was likely that Barbara's younger brother felt more responsibility for his elder sister since their father had died. He, like Sarah's brother, had become 'wise ones' (Goffman, 1963).

When looking at the findings through gender lenses, men appeared to be almost as involved in 'care' as women in providing companionship, interpreting skills, help through crises and transitions. This support was rarely asked for or negotiated, but occurred as a result of the development of informal coping strategies by kin who were concerned about the quality of life of their hearing impaired relative. Although further research is needed, it may be that men are involved to an unexpected degree because what they provide does not feel like traditional 'tending' care to them, but rather like some form of communication.

Summary

Hearing impaired people in this study found support in a wide variety of social relations with their kin. The most successful appeared to involve some sort of reciprocal arrangement. There was also a strong unpredictable element in the kinship patterns especially among sisters.

A major difficulty confronting the kin investigated was the problem of interpreting and understanding the ambiguous nature of the needs of their hearing impaired relations, and consequently being able to provide appropriate care. In most cases hearing impaired people themselves did not have the confidence or desire to explain their communication requirements in detail even if they understood them. It was felt that sharing such details did not belong with their kin, but more with spouses or voluntary friends where there was more genuine affection.

The reluctance of hearing impaired elderly people to be more explicit about their needs may be partly explained by their awareness that they run counter to prevailing domestic norms in many English families. While it is not necessarily always the case, feelings of 'belonging' and 'cohesion' have traditionally been generated orally and indirectly through the easy sharing of domestic sociability in a way in which hearing impaired people can not join. Repetition is therefore needed. However, here is where the paradoxical heart of the problem emerges. It may be that in the context in which these people lived, social norms dictated that these so called trivial conversations with unstated meaning are not considered important enough for repetition. As we have seen, it is extremely difficult for hearing impaired people not to feel that it is they who are unimportant, and they can become caught 'between two worlds': those who hear and those who do not.

There is then a strong case for education and counselling to help families expand their understanding of appropriate responses so that care and concern for their hearing impaired kin is expressed more effectively. Hearing impaired people themselves also have the responsibility to learn to lip-read and to increase their skills in reading nonverbal cues and body language. Without these interventions, the present community care policy where families play such an important part, will be of limited value for elderly hearing impaired people.

On the whole women seemed slightly more involved in supporting their hearing impaired relations than men, although men were much in evidence either as 'watch dogs' or in direct help through repetition, interpretation, companionship etc.

Generally if kin relationships were unsatisfactory before the hearing impairment, they remained so afterwards. There were no examples of the hearing loss 'cementing' a formerly uncertain relationship.

Evidence provided by the hearing impaired people in this book suggested that geographical distance from kin could act as a communication challenge rather than a barrier provided relationships had been strong before the distance existed. The next chapter will complete the social network picture by focusing on wider networks including friendships, professionals and religious involvement.

CHAPTER 9

Wider networks

Introduction

Having considered kinship, we now explore the impact of hearing impairment on friendship, relationships with professional helpers and associational groups, amongst them churches. In doing this, it is important to remember that categories such as these are not mutually exclusive: there were examples of kin who were also friends and professionals.

Abrams argues that beyond close kin, 'our strongest bases of informal social care are those of non-located moral communities associated with churches, races, friendship groups and certain occupational groups – not neighbourhoods' (1980: 16).

It will be suggested that hearing impaired people have considerable difficulty establishing or mobilizing a social network of friends because of the communication barriers which their hearing difficulties are likely to present, as there is a basic note of dissonance between the voluntary nature of friendship and the implications of being hearing impaired.

We will analyse these difficulties using Unger and Powell's (1980) three levels of social network formation: the first level is the nuclear family, close friends and relatives; second, neighbours, more distant friends and relatives and certain service providers; and third, the still less intimate defined by superficial or infrequent contact often in the context of social institutions.

Within this model, there will be an analysis of old and new friendships, responsibility for network formation, the two primary strategies needed when conversing with a hearing people specifically 'looking' and 'repeating', and the role of helping professionals generally.

Lastly in an expansion of our understanding of the third level of social support, there is a discussion as an example, of the role which church involvement has had in the lives of its hearing impaired members with a specific focus on tradition, fellowship versus solitude, the inductive loop system and belonging, and the support of the clergyman and his church.

The specific nature of friendship will first be discussed. The ambiguity surrounding this concept requires a comprehensive discussion to help to capture its core meaning.

The nature of friendship

The conventional definition of friendship is that of a freely chosen, voluntary and predominantly expressive relationship (Cohen and Rajkowski, 1982). While there are certain norms and conventions which pattern friends' behaviour towards one another (Suttles, 1970), friendship of itself is not seen as being incorporated into the institutional fabric of society in the way that kinship is. Certainly, not all societies foster or tolerate the freedom and flexibility that is a typical feature of British friendship.

Within the literature, some attempt has been made to define an idealized version of friendship sometimes known as 'genuine', 'real' or 'true' friendship. In these ideal friendships, the solidarity of friends, based solely on their personal and voluntary commitment to each other, is taken to be unfettered by any selfish or instrumental concerns. From this perspective, such friendship can be recognized as a bond of enormous moral significance, as one of the highest expressions of voluntary altruistic commitment there can be between people (Brain, 1976).

The literature, however, makes the point that such ideal relationships are rare and may more nearly resemble a concept of 'best friends'. The pattern usually found is a range of relationships which combine in different ways the various elements that are entailed in the general notion of friendship. This appears to be the case not only in straightforward behaviour terms (for example, when friends meet and the types of activities undertaken), but also with respect to the level of intimacy, trust, and commitment experienced.

Despite the complexity surrounding the concept of friendship, it is agreed that it is a voluntary relationship in that the ties are chosen quite freely and may be ended as desired. Friendship is, on the other hand, often a little less free than it appears. For example, many friendships originate between people who are involved with each other in formal organizations of some sort, which have some effect on shaping their ties. However, the extent to which they will recognize their relationship as one of friendship will depend in part on the extent to which they see them as free of organizational constraints.

Finally, one of the foremost features of friendship is that it is essentially a relationship of equality. In other words, in addition to being informal and free from broader structural imperatives, friendship is a bond in which issues of hierarchy and authority have no bearing. Therefore, it would be expected that the majority of friendships occur between people who occupy broadly similar social positions. There is of course, nothing within the notion of friendship itself that requires this to be so, but the economic and social divisions within the society certainly encourage it. In other words friends are normally of roughly the same age and class position. They also tend to share similar domestic circumstances, to be of the same gender, to have similar ethnic backgrounds and, where it is of social consequence, to belong to the same religion (Lazarsfeld and Merton, 1954).

We will now explore how having a disability in the family may make an impact on friendship development specifically in the formation of a social network.

Disability: the three levels of social support reviewed

Unger and Powell (1980) suggest there is a need for three levels of social support when there is disability in the family. Although each of the levels overlaps with the next, these differing degrees of intimacy require somewhat different interpersonal skills. For example, the first level of support, the nuclear family, close friends and relations, relies on what has been called the consensual norm, while the second level of support, neighbours and more distant friends and relations, is based more on a norm of reciprocity. The third level of support is more distant and may rely on institutional or professional obligations.

The next section will focus on the first level of social support with reference to close friendships.

Hearing impairment and old and new friendship

Acquired hearing loss especially of a severe or profound degree, is likely to make one lose some friendships (Elliott, 1978). The people in this study in fact presented a much more complex picture, suggesting that additional psychosocial factors were operating, specifically gender, class and personality.

Sam, deafened at 17, was the one person in the study who believed he had lost friends, and wished he had more in the present. He recalled:

> [when] friends come to visit, ... they ... talk to Julia [as they are her friends] ... I will ... talk to perhaps one other person ... [in the group], ... [the topic of our discussion] might not be the same as everyone else is talking about.

Undoubtedly Sam's shy personality and profound hearing loss had slowed down his ability to make friends and limited his pleasure, but there were also other factors. First, Sam and Julia had moved to their present house from the North only two years ago. Moves are well known for disrupting social networks and are especially difficult to rebuild if one is hearing impaired (Sainsbury, 1986; Holmes and Rahe, 1967). Meeting strangers can be a particularly uncomfortable task since one's social skills often feel depleted (Beattie, 1981). Sam recalled:

> I had more and better friends at Leeds University where people didn't 'pigeon hole' you as they do in my present job. They were more open minded there ... perhaps the [university atmosphere] helped.

Sam felt that his present work environment was not conducive to his growth intellectually in the way of a stimulating career or emotionally through involvement with colleagues/friends. An aborted friendship with a deaf colleague, had confirmed that differences beyond the common factor of deafness could be too great. These experiences contrasted sharply with pleasurable times he recalled with members of his Sub-Aqua club at Leeds:

> I particularly enjoyed my friends in the diving club ... it wasn't so much the common interest, but the fact that we all drank together afterwards ... I don't feel I have that sort of experience ... [now].

Sam was able to transcend both his shyness and deafness by the 'warming up' process of drinking in a pub. The pub atmosphere was likely to feel more congenial because of his working class roots.

Gender was another factor as Sam believed it was much easier to make new acquaintances with women rather than men. He recalled:

> With ... women especially, I can understand what they are saying even if they ... don't know I am deaf; ... I don't think a man has as much patience as a woman ... perhaps it's not just patience ... it's more understanding of the other person.

However, deafened people have other requirements for effective communication and Julia gave an example:

> [While] a woman will get more upset or angry if you don't understand the first time, ... a man is likely not to be so bothered by [having to repeat] ... Remember ... John? He used to talk to you a lot,..[and] I never once saw him get angry or impatient ... [at having] to repeat himself ...

Sam then recalled his friendship with John more fully:

> in Leeds, I ... shared a house with a friend and his wife ... [John,] would talk to me, and it never bothered him if I misunderstood something ... [He would] ... either repeat it or explain it in a different way ...

Not only did John have a high toleration for repetition perhaps having some appreciation of it's helpfulness in a more general sense (Tannen, 1989), he had also acquired the art of paraphrasing. Thus Sam's current isolation was not because of lack of effort as he circulated widely. For example, recently he had enrolled in a French class, helped a friend restore his cottage in France, and taken part in a sailing club for the disabled. He had no desire to go to a Deaf club although he had attended them in the past and even taught at a school for Deaf children.

Sam had discovered that he was 'too hearing' in his thinking to feel comfortable in the Deaf community (Harvey, 1989). Also, living with Julia who was both hearing and middle class, meant that she took charge of their social life by writing letters, making telephone calls, and interpreting in social situations. Sam recalled:

> I used to write to ... [family and friends] when I was at college on my own, but ... I've let it drift and I don't write very much.

Julia may have colluded with Sam in creating his social dependence, but it was certainly not intentional. Julia simply saw her social skills as a reflection of her gender (Tannen, 1991) and that the process of what I call Developing Mutually Enhancing Networks (DMEN) was a sensible strategy for everyone, hearing or deaf, as it guarded against emotional isolation and intellectual stagnation. Despite their many moves, Julia and Sam's joint network had in fact become quite extensive consisting of over forty relatives and friends when formalized on paper.

With this couple, the factors of personality type, class background and gender were more significant than deafness in causing Sam's personal isolation. He had assimilated enough into the middle-class hearing world to make a certain peace with it (Glickman, 1986).

Joy found herself in a similar situation to Sam's. However, she had been more successful in holding on to her old friends. This was largely possible because she and her husband, Mike, unlike Sam, had returned to their childhood home. She recalled:

> I've kept all the friends I went to school with ... [those since we got married] ...
> and then there's all the [new] friends around ... since we've moved [back] ...

Despite her working-class roots, Joy adopted what might be called a middle-class manner of relating, for example old friends were substitutes for kin (Willmott, 1986). Contrary to what might be expected (Beattie, 1981), Joy's experiences suggested that hearing loss need not deplete one's social skills. The fact that she was able to pick up with old friendships in an easy manner implicitly revealed that she was known to have the qualities of a good friend. She explained:

> Some ... friends ... I've made since I've been deaf ... As a matter of fact, [I'm
> going] to my friend's place tonight ... I was around last week and before ... we
> went out on a Saturday ... I made [these] friends, .. not Mike, ... he didn't know
> them.

Autonomy in friendship making and maintaining was very important to Joy. As people going through identity and life changes (Askham, 1984), as well as those who are suddenly disabled, specifically deafened (Sloss Luey, 1980), do lose friends, it was of particular interest to see how Joy kept hers. She appeared unconscious of any strategy. She remembered:

> I had to tell ... [my old friends] to speak slowly, please; and I suppose they see how Mike speaks to me, and they do the same ... they can see that I am still the same person ...

Because Joy had an understanding husband and loyal old friends, she could build on these relationships and go on to establish new friendships. Also Joy had no difficulty making appropriate disclosures about her deafness. She actually appeared to be informing or educating her old friends rather than 'disclosing'. Her skill might have been a reflection of the fact that she was completely free from any sense of shame connected to her sudden loss of hearing (Wax, 1989), none the less, she did feel a certain sense of devalued status sometimes connected with being a member of a minority group (Vernon and Makowsky, 1969).

As people with acquired hearing loss generally already have established marriages, families, careers, leisure and social activities, it follows they would be inclined to maintain these life styles (Neugarten, 1972). While some people experiencing traumatic hearing loss might have to go through a period of isolation and withdrawal, closely associated with grieving, Joy avoided this behaviour and continued in her easy capacity to keep and sustain friendships. Nevertheless, she did not always meet with success. Mike recalled:

> it all depends whether other people are willing to make the effort ... some people won't, ... [like] Pat over the road ... [she and her husband] are nice enough people ... they'll say good morning and all that, but they won't say much else to Joy ...

Mike pinpointed what appeared to be a classic encounter between a hearing and deaf person (Higgens, 1980). He saw the problem as one of embarrassment in that their neighbour didn't know how to talk to Joy. We do not know what was behind this neighbour's anti-social behaviour, but Joy had her own opinion:

> there are always some people ... that just can't accept ... and they've no idea how to ... talk to me ... [Pat] won't talk to me when I'm alone ...

Joy admittedly had some frustrating encounters with neighbours as confirmed by Sainsbury (1986). Like Sam, she discovered there were compensations specifically in cross-gender relationships. Possibly cross-gender friendships are a particular feature of couple friendships when one partner has been deafened provided the couples involved have acquired the security and mutual understanding with one another to allow for its development.

Sussman (1986) suggests that a trait of people who have come to terms with their hearing loss is their capacity to socialize with other hearing impaired people. Although both Joy and Sam had links with NADP (National Association for Deafened People), neither claimed a good friendship with another couple like themselves. This may have left Joy and Mike with a certain sensitivity about their life being particularly hard. For example, Joy recalled:

> We don't know any other deaf couples so we can't compare their [situation with ours] ... we know plenty of hearing people, but obviously it is different since they can communicate a lot easier than we can.

Returning to Julia and Sam, Julia's calm organized approach towards her and Sam's social network was a direct contrast to the more anxious attitudes of some of the hearing wives in the study. In the following section, an attempt will be made to consider their concerns.

Social networks: whose responsibility?

The study produced three hearing wives who were anxious about their responsibility for 'social network' formation. The most articulate was Joe's second wife, Sarah. As we have seen, Joe's early attempts at developing a social network were thwarted by his own kin and then by his first wife.

Now Sarah wished to help him by explaining her understanding of the term which focused on friendship for relaxation and intimacy more than sociability. While it is possible to have both, there was the implicit suggestion that the gentleness of Sarah's feminine network appeared to be more appropriate for Joe at this time while he was gradually breaking free from his former isolated marginal lifestyle (Wax, 1989). Joe, on the other hand, was mildly resistant to this arrangement as it was 'women's talk' (Tannen, 1991).

To a certain extent, Joe had compensated for his isolation by becoming a workaholic. Because Joe had lost his wife and sons through divorce, his sister through mental illness and his parents through death, it seemed that for a time he lost trust in close relationships generally as they had only brought him sorrow. Although Joe was appreciative and admiring of all Sarah's efforts to build a friendship circle, he was also aware that his enjoyment level was not quite 'in tune' with hers. Joe explained his attitude:

> My idea of a dinner party is conversation [not nattering], ... that you talk about things, ... but when your hearing aid is just picking up other people's talking ... which makes it difficult to concentrate on your next door neighbour, ... it gets a bit frustrating.

Joe's deafness meant that he could not converse at Sarah's supper parties in the manner that he would have liked, but also he was disappointed in the general tone of the conversations that he could hear because topics of 'true' consequence were not discussed.

Regardless of Sarah's success in DMEN (Developing Mutually Enhancing Networks), she continued to be anxious at what she considered to be Joe's dependence on her for his social life as she was unaware that husbands are often dependent on their wives in this way even when they have perfect hearing (Allan, 1989). Gwen, Arthur's wife, also had a strong sense of responsibility concerning their mutual social network. Like Sarah, she had no experience of men's social networks, for example, she did not understand why Arthur did not need a 'best friend' in the way she did. Arthur, like Sam from a working-class background, found his friendships in his 'mates', which were context based. Gwen was able to acknowledge that her anxious attitude about Arthur's friends was more in connection with her own fear of taking friendship risks. Nevertheless, this sense of responsibility gave her additional courage to do things which she might not have done otherwise.

As a bicultural couple, Gwen and Arthur's social network was drawn from both Deaf and hearing communities. Although a larger catchment area, integration had to be worked at gently, but was eventually successful on both sides as a result of the quality of Gwen's friends, her personal sensitivity, and her skill at Signing. Arthur's easy intelligence, lip-reading skill, and charming manner also helped to break the ice. However, both knew how easy it was to cause offence when the wrong thing was said or done. Gwen related:

> we know a couple much older than us who are in [the] Break Through [Trust] ... [Sheila's] partially hearing ... [and Jack's] a teacher of the Deaf ... If there is a problem,...[Jack's] there ironing it out, ... [for example], we had a 'skittles' evening and there was a problem over money for the coffee, so [Jack] paid for it himself ... and said, 'Oh well, we don't want to give Deaf people a bad name.'

Arthur and Gwen believed that Jack's apparent kindness was actually motivated by a fear that his image and that of his companions would be tarnished by the stereotype of Deaf people being childish and irresponsible.

Gwen, however, went further than Sarah or Jack in understanding that what their deaf partners really wanted were friendships based upon equality, whether with themselves or other hearing people. Because of the very nature of the disability, this is difficult to achieve unless the adjustments necessary are seen in a new light. We will discuss this aspect of the problem in the next section.

Revisioning the adjustments required by hearing people: looking and repeating

If people with acquired hearing loss are to be perceived as 'different' and 'equal', a revisioning process has to take place. It has already begun in the Deaf community as linguists have given Sign language a new respectability, proclaiming it to be a genuine language with its own syntax (Sacks, 1990).

While people with acquired hearing loss do not require those who hear to learn a new language, they do require cooperation so that lip-reading can take place. This cooperation is about making themselves truly accessible to relaxed communication with people with acquired hearing loss. While there are many factors that could be explored here, certain key factors have emerged in this study as being the most helpful in the communication exchange.

As we have seen, hearing impaired people need the ETTA (Effort, Time, Thought and Attention) required so that a relaxed conversation can begin. For a conversation to continue and a relationship to develop, two other important interactive processes will have emerged: 'looking' and 'repeating'. For relaxed communication to flourish, these two processes need to be seen in a fresh light.

Sociologists (Allan, 1989), social psychologists (Noller, 1984) and linguists (Tannen, 1991) suggest that 'looking' or gaze behaviour facilitates the development of intimate relationships generally. There is clear evidence for a looking-liking connection of the following type:

> the more you look at me [the more attention you give me], the more I will like you.

This connection is confirmed in Ellyson's (1978) study which shows a correlation between 'looking' behaviour and husbands who are well adjusted in their marriages. Ellyson observes that these husbands both looked and listened to their wives when their wives spoke to them. The 'looking' behaviour is seen to be a reflection of the husbands' desire to understand rather than control their wives. This finding implies that the 'looking behaviour' required as a communication strategy for people with acquired hearing loss, does in fact facilitate intimate relationships more generally.

In a similar way, 'repetition' has been discovered to be of greater value than conventionally understood (Ree, 1999). Tannen (1989) argues that 'repetition' is a pervasive, fundamental, infinitely useful conversational strategy; it has varied purposes, for example production, comprehension, connection and interaction. In addition, it gives poetry its rhythmical character and has in fact been highly valued and studied in literary texts. Gertrude Stein said:

> Repeating then is in every one, in every one in their being and their feeling and their way of realising everything ... (Stein, 1935: 214)

Resistance would be expected to requests for behaviour change along with the above interpretation of 'looking' and 'repeating' and the conceptualization of ETTA. There is also a cultural dimension in that English people have not been known for putting their energy into intimate, emotional and personal communication (Paxman, 1998). However, for hearing impaired people themselves and their hopes for friendships built upon equality and reciprocity, these conceptualizations suggest a way of transforming the perceived caring obligatory aspect of communication with them into something of greater value and interest.

Since this chapter has touched on the attitudes of professionals, it is appropriate to explore the role of professionals in more depth.

Professionals and service providers: how helpful?

The discussion now focuses on Unger and Powell's second level of support for families where there is a disability. This level contains neighbours, more distant friends and relatives and selected professionals and service providers. Research suggests that families where there is a disabled member tend to use medical and other formal support services as much as other families, but they tend not to utilize them to a degree consistent with their level of need (McAllister *et al.*, 1973).

In looking at the specific professional–client relationship, Appleton and Minchom (1991) describe the professional–client models which are used when working with children and their families. Here they have been adapted for professionals working with clients who are disabled. They are called the 'expert model', the 'consumer rights model', the 'social network/systems model', and the 'empowerment model'. As the latter will be the most relevant in the 1990s, it will be described. The 'empowerment model' has three main tenets. First, professionals actively promote their clients' sense of control over decisions affecting them. Secondly, they are sensitive to the rights of clients to opt into the professional system at a level they choose; and lastly, professionals must be sensitive to the unique adaptational style that each family and social network employs. These three tenets are not a blueprint since each family is unique. However, their focus on service quality and consumer control is representative of the empowerment approach which is now believed to be crucial in the long term for promoting emotional growth and a responsible attitude in both clients and professionals.

The evidence of this present study was that there was a wide range of professional help available to people. It varied not only in its specific nature, but also in its effectiveness. Some excellent sensitive help was offered alongside help which was felt to be ineffective and unsatisfactory. There were also examples of attempted help which was destructive.

Doctors

Contrary to expectation, people who received the worst treatment from doctors did not necessarily feel the most anger towards them. Two profoundly deaf men perceived that they had actually been deafened by drugs prescribed for them by doctors. Nevertheless, neither appeared to be harbouring great bitterness because of it. Sam remembered:

> About four months before I became deaf, I had an infection in my ear. I went to the doctor to see about it and I had an injection to clear up the infection ... the infection cleared up. After that I started to experience giddy spells with the room going round and round and then quite suddenly I became deaf in the left ear. Then gradually over a period of time, ... I became deaf in the right ear ... When I became deaf in the left ear which was very sudden, I went back to the doctor [who] had a quick look in my ear and sent me straight to the Ear Nose and Throat Hospital to see the specialist and they said they might be able to do something ...

At first Sam and his mother like many others, were hopeful for a cure (Jones, Kyle and Wood, 1987). However, after further tests, Sam recalled he was told:

> 'there's nothing we can do about it; sorry about all that', but I think the cause was drug toxicity [from the injection I received for the infection]. I can't prove anything now.

This first experience along with subsequent experiences since had left Sam feeling:

> Well, I don't think I've had much help from doctors in the medical profession ... the impression I get from them is that if they cannot do anything, ... they are not interested. They'd rather deal with people they can have more success with ...

Sam's partner, Julia, spoke more forcefully against the doctor who had treated Sam expressing her belief that it was only Sam's amazing fortitude which had carried him through the experience so well. Nigerian Anthony had a similar initial experience; but eventually, perhaps partly because he was a doctor himself, he had received excellent care at the hands of the medical profession in that grants were found for his complete rehabilitation.

Study participants also mentioned difficulties with doctors concerning the diagnosis of deafness. In one case there was a misdiagnosis. Martha related:

> No, I blame the doctor that attended me [then]. I was seven or eight ... it was during the war [when] I had scarlet fever ... which was very rare ... and the doctor thought it was tonsillitis.

It may be that the outcome of Martha's illness at that time in history would have been the same; however, in Martha's eyes, a doctor had made a mistake from which she had suffered. There were other people in the study who recalled their doctor's insensitivity at the time of diagnosis. Deafened Joy remembered how her doctor presented her with a piece of paper on which he had written her irreversible condition, at a time when she was unsupported. Mike, her husband, remembered his own feelings:

> when Joy was first in hospital ... the surgeon told me that there was no possibility of ... [her hearing] ever coming back again ... At that particular time, it did really upset me ...

Mike and Joy had a mixed experience with their medical care. Many years later Joy was pleased with the quality of care she received during and after her cochlear implant operation. Barbara also had a mixed experience. Currently, she was pleased with her GP who was open and direct and did not patronize. Previously, she had been less fortunate in seeing an ENT consultant who had doubted her word when she told him her degree of deafness until he was presented with her audiogram, at which time he apologized.

Joe and Anne's medical care had been more satisfactory. Anne found her ENT consultant helpful when she was thinking through whether or not she wished to wear a hearing aid as she felt that he treated her as an adult capable of making wise choices. Joe benefited from his doctor's interest which assisted him in meeting his second wife.

Another way of exploring the quality of the relationship between hearing impaired people and the medical profession is through an analysis of their experiences with regard to acquiring hearing aids. With reference to Unger and Powell's model, this process of hearing aid acquisition takes place on the third level of more distant professional relationships specifically those based in social/medical institutions.(Schilling, Gilchrist and Schinke, 1984). We will now explore this process as a social policy issue as it currently takes place within the National Health Service.

The process of hearing aid distribution: a social policy issue?

People's feelings about their hearing aids are complex. Undoubtedly there is some connection with how people feel about them and how they are actually treated when fitted with one. Although patients may see their ENT consultant or his resident on special request, they usually encounter hearing aid technicians who service and distribute the aids and batteries. They perform a very useful service, but additional information is difficult to obtain. The professor in this study made an attempt to find out some basic information about his acquired hearing loss. He was met with the following reply by the technician:

> Oh you'll have to get a letter from your doctor, we can't tell you this ... that's the way we do things.

This reply irritated and angered Frank, who was joined by other people in the study in making the point that the patient at the bottom of the NHS bureaucratic structure felt depersonalized when attending the ENT clinic. As it happened, Frank in his capacity as a university administrator, was able to address his complaint to the former Dean of a London medical school who happened to be chairing one of the many meetings which Frank attended. Frank bluntly stated:

> I think most of the medical men treat their patients as if they are 'morons' you know.

The Dean defended his profession by saying:

> Well, different patients react differently. Some really don't want to know the details about what's wrong with them: others want to know with precision when in fact we can't give a precise diagnosis.

The Dean appeared insensitive to the destructive effect caused by the indiscriminate use of the blanket policy of nondisclosure. People wanted to understand their condition and did not feel that 'a label' was sufficient. This suggests that information and rehabilitation counselling would have been more appropriate (Kyle, Jones and Wood, 1985). Even if they did not want hearing aids, all the people in this study wanted to know the facts about their or their partner's condition and some went to considerable lengths to discover them.

This suggests that the implications for social policy are twofold: doctors as part of their training generally need to learn firstly to assess their patients' resources for coping with 'loss'. As part of this assessment, doctors need to learn to speak the truth as they perceive it gently and directly; and in doing this, they need to trust their patients to mobilize the resources they require to manage what is told to them.

Secondly, although not a straightforward matter (May, 1992), doctors need to develop a deeper understanding of their therapeutic function in relation to their hearing impaired patients (Balint, 1965). They may do this specifically by being honest with themselves and their patients about their own limitations. This means that they have to trust themselves and their patients to resolve their initial feelings of disappointment in discovering the doctor's fallibility in not having a cure for deafness. In most cases doctors are intelligent, dedicated, and skilled human beings, but they also have diagnostic, therapeutic, professional and personal limitations. If the patients are allowed to see their doctors struggle, it could help them come to terms with their own limitations.

These findings therefore suggest that a more discriminating and enlightened social policy in the manner of distributing hearing aids would be of significant help in transforming the patients' attitudes to their disability, and its specific symbol, the hearing aid. This policy could be implemented by doctors being taught to be more 'open' with their patients, treating them in a more adult manner and being aware of psychosocial issues.

Arthur, the person in the study originating from the Deaf community, believed it was not just doctors who had ill used their influence. The focus now shifts to Arthur's specific views about other professionals.

Other professionals: can the legacy of the past be transformed?

Arthur began by explaining his view:

> I am always suspicious of the motives of professionals who work with Deaf people, two professions in particular ... doctors and teachers ... are strongly

anti-sign language. For hundreds of years, sign language was not used in Deaf schools. I think the teachers and the doctors were in the forefront in that they could tell the parents that the child should not Sign, that they should only talk, and no waving hands around. They would be fitted with hearing aids so in that way oral communication became more dominant,..[as] parents of deaf children would only listen to the professionals, ... they would not listen to deaf people because none of them had met deaf people before ...

Arthur's partner, Gwen, had a slightly different perspective. She thought that misleading Deaf people (Wax, 1989) could be the result of inexperience and that sometimes professionals knew their knowledge or the system were inadequate, but had no idea how to improve it. Arthur and Gwen were unanimous in their belief that social workers were ineffective when interacting with Deaf people. Arthur said:

I suppose a lot of these social workers like being with deaf adults, ... but they tend to see deaf people as being like deaf children needing help, ... at least social workers do far less harm because the harm has been done anyway when the children were small ...

Arthur stressed the fact that social workers have tended to maintain rather than radically transform a HCD (Hearing Construction of Deafness) (Harris, 1995). As we have seen, this is a negative conception of deafness which contrasts with a more positive conception held by members of the Deaf community or DCD (the Deaf Construction of Deafness). Arthur recalled:

I used to go to Deaf clubs ... I am not a member any more ... it was the way these clubs were ... run ... to my mind, ... [the social workers] see these Deaf clubs as part of their fiefdom.

Gwen wished to balance Arthur's perspective, but she also alluded to HCD (Hearing Construction of Deafness). She said:

[this situation] is not so much now as in the old days ... a lot of professionals seemed to think there is something wrong with the deaf person that has to be put right ...

Although aware of all these injustices, Arthur acknowledged the responsibility of Deaf people in transforming the HCD. He said:

I think Deaf people themselves do not help by relying on the social workers for help, ... [and] in many ways ... social workers subconsciously encourage [dependency] ... [in order] to safeguard their jobs ... that's my opinion ...

Arthur's point of the 'needy helper' of Deaf people is well supported in the counselling literature. Corker (1994) succeeds in creating a useful typology of needy counsellors, of these, 'the benevolent humanitarian' is the one that exemplifies Arthur's specific point.

Gwen appeared concerned that Arthur did not mix his rhetoric with reality. She focused on the social worker who currently visited them:

> Ours is all right, ... It's an automatic thing ... 'deaf' ... you get on the books of the social worker ... [it would be] better for those who [really] need it.

Arthur added:

> The one in this area is very good – he won't see you unless you want to see him.

Neither Gwen nor Arthur understood here that having a social worker today is a completely voluntary matter. Because most local authorities are understaffed, Gwen was correct in assuming that the need was greater elsewhere. It would appear that their social worker or deafness worker had adopted the model of 'information/link' which Parrott suggests may be the model of the future (1992).

Throughout this discussion, Arthur refused to claim a definite cultural identity for himself as other members of the Deaf community have done (Lane, 1984). Like others, he focused on the acceptance of BSL as the way forward to accepting Deaf people as 'the act of Signing itself has become a declaration of political affiliation' (Harris, 1995: 157).

Although members of the Deaf community may now be operating with these criteria, the situation is far more complex than Arthur presented. There are many people who might like to learn BSL for one reason or other, but find it too difficult, as for example Arthur's own parents' in-law, Beatrice and Andrew. Conversely, severely hearing impaired Henry (40), talked about his feeling of liberation when he first began Signing classes:

> I felt I was in a straight jacket before I learned BSL ... at first I was terrified of using it ... The tutor [called it taking] 'a sacred vow with which to overcome your inhibition'. In other words, it doesn't matter what people think ... [as long as it's] 'OK' for yourself.

While Henry obviously benefited from BSL, in that it helped him to adopt a more positive identity or Deaf Construction of Deafness (DCD) (Harris, 1995), it was less useful for other members in this study. Despite the fact that they had the same degree of hearing loss as Henry and Arthur, their identification with the hearing world was stronger, and they had made a certain peace with the communication strategies already available to them.

One group of professionals which Arthur did not condemn for their misuse of authority was the clergy. Religion, implicitly if not explicitly, was an important aspect of Arthur and Gwen's life, and for this reason they chose a church wedding. A chaplain of the Deaf married them and the service itself was done in English and BSL. The next section will focus on what other people in the study felt about the support which their faith, or involvement with a community church gave them.

Religious involvement

Church membership, like some other associational groups, allows the suspension or realignment of the expectations of reciprocity and mutual exchange on which friendship and neighbouring usually depend (Bulmer, 1987). This may be one of the reasons why historically church membership has been particularly important for prelingually deaf people (Sainsbury, 1986).

In continuing with the third level of social support (Unger and Powell, 1980), study participants represented a wide range of feelings and experiences with regard to their personal faith and more formal commitment to church attendance, worship and fellowship. Although the practices of the people here can not be generalized to the total population because of the small numbers involved, some interesting evidence emerged. For example, as many as nine of the 27 people studied here were regular attenders of a church or synagogue, six were occasional attenders, five were episodic and seven were what might be called visitors. Despite the fact that it was difficult to hear in many churches since loop systems had yet to be installed, although this is slowly improving, the people in the study still went and regular attendance was actually 17 per cent higher than found in the population at large (Brierley, 1991). Four factors which may be important in explaining this are tradition, fellowship versus solitude, loop systems and belonging, and the clergyman as support.

Tradition

A number of people in the study based their decision to be involved with a church on the tradition of their families, that is it is part of their heritage. Arthur and Gwen, from strict Church of Scotland backgrounds, talked about their decision to be married in church rather than to cohabit or be married in a register office. Arthur explained:

> I think it was sort of a deeper instinct ... partly religious tradition. That sort of thing ... [is taken] very seriously in Scotland. If for example, people lived together on the Isle of Lewis in the Hebrides [where Gwen's family come from], they'd be shunned.

Gwen agreed:

> It's conditioning ... family and other sorts of ties ... religious partly, cultural ... well I don't come from an environment where people live together ...

Arthur and Gwen were only too aware of the stigma which accompanied deafness. Because of their close family ties, they did not wish to risk causing offence and further stigmatizing themselves by living together before marriage.

Fellowship versus solitude

The people in the study varied in how much fellowship they hoped for when attending a place of worship. One hard of hearing woman of 84, Theo, attended an evangelical chapel. She described her experience:

> I take my Bible and the person [who] sits next to me ... finds the place if I don't hear, ... immediately ... [I] have a friend [who] looks after me.

While Theo was able to experience the helpfulness of others in church, severely hearing impaired Joe, who regularly attended synagogue, found the greatest satisfaction from just being at peace rather than in relating to others. In contrast, his Gentile wife, Sarah, enjoyed socializing in the synagogue for its own sake. Beatrice, Gwen's mother, experienced a deeper kind of social support from her church network.

These examples illustrate the capacity of each individual to find what they needed in church or synagogue experiences. However, some people in the study experienced deep frustration in connection with church attendance. Severely deaf Henry, aged 40, had particular difficulties. Whereas he and his wife were both studying for the Ministry, Henry suffered greatly whenever he attended the fellowship hour in the church hall after the service. This was because he desperately wanted to relate to others, but felt helpless because the 'background noise' made his hearing aids useless. Kay, his wife, described a row they had after a Sunday service:

> I thought [after the teapot lid had broken and Henry had been upset] that [he] was just resenting ... that I'd been in the limelight [preaching] at church, but he said distraughtly: 'I don't know anybody there ... nobody talks to me'.

Kay reflected further:

> Once I realized that ... [Henry] was feeling isolated with so many people, ... and nobody talking to him ... and Clive ... [our son] misbehaving, ... and also the business about our [uncertain] future ... and just general tiredness which Henry's been feeling, ... a combination of things, ... [then] the tension disappeared and we were able to calm down and ... meet. But sometimes there are just sort of misunderstandings.

With not even his wife truly supporting him, it was understandable that Henry should feel isolated and helpless, unable to get out from underneath his inspirational image, and unable to clarify his needs in an adult way (van Dongen-Garrad, 1983).

This illustration points to the domino effect which could result when there is no strategy for helping a severely hearing impaired parishioner integrate into the church's fellowship hour. In this particular case, lines of responsibility for this process were unclear. Once Kay understood how Henry was feeling, it was their joint responsibility to explain the problem to her vicar or someone on the staff of the theological college which Henry attended so that helpful strategies could be formulated. Although those in authority might be unfamiliar with the specific needs of hearing impaired people, they could listen.

In the second instance, as Henry became more confident, he needed to be more open about his need for clarification, and for taking time off when he got tired and felt stressed.

The final step is for the implementation of a mutually formulated integration strategy. This subject cannot be dealt with adequately here, although it is possible to make a start. For example, on days when Kay was to preach, someone could volunteer to help Henry with the children thus freeing him to concentrate on lip-reading parishioners. He could be encouraged to meet members of the congregation in their homes where the atmosphere is usually more relaxed and he would be able to use his hearing aids. This would mean when Henry did meet people in the more formal setting of the church hall, he could build upon a relationship that had already begun rather than meeting a complete stranger with unknown lip patterns.

The inductive loop system and belonging

The inductive loop system is the most common device installed in churches to aid hearing impaired people. A 'magnetic field' is produced by running a circuit of wire around a room which plugs into an amplifier, part of the sound system. The sound is received by the hearing impaired person with no background noise provided they have a 'pick up coil' in their hearing aids which most aids now have. The effect is threefold: the sound comes directly from the microphone into the ear rather than from some far off loudspeaker making the sound clearer and less distorted, volume can be individually adjusted, and all background noises from sources outside the loop are eliminated (Boone, 1993).

All churches do not have loop systems which work adequately if they manage to have one at all. Max, an elderly widower, was not one of the fortunate ones. Although he had lived a full and rich life as a husband, father, teacher, headmaster and once President of the National Union of Teachers, he now found himself unable to hear in his local church. He said:

> I used to go up to this church, All Saints, ... but I don't go now ... not because I have any difference of [religious] view, ... but I can't sit in that church and ... hear a good sermon! ... I know that's not the only thing you go to church for, but I can't hear a single sentence, ... it's a lovely church ... and I like to go, ... but it doesn't seem worthwhile.

Max's example was representative of the problems caused when elderly intelligent people are cut off prematurely from the stimulating aspect of faith because they cannot hear the preaching. The question must then be asked, 'Who is it who speaks up for hearing impaired people and their needs in the local churches?' Although various groups have begun to campaign for the rights of hearing impaired people (for example, the Hard of Hearing Christian Fellowship), the established Church of England has barely begun to address this problem. This was evidenced by the fact that in the 150 page report entitled (Ageing, 1990) drawn up by the Church of England's Social Policy Committee of the Board for Social Responsibility, there was no mention of hearing impairment.

The clergyman and his church as support

A theme that ran through people's comments on Church involvement was its importance in times of trouble, special occasions, and status transitions. Deafened Sam and his partner, Julia, talked about their experience. Julia said:

> I go sometimes ... only ... [Sam] ... [doesn't] come with me. It's boring ... [he] can't hear anything. I like songs at Christmas time ... I like to go to the Carol services.

Although Julia can hear perfectly, it was really only the Christmas music which drew her to church. She also admitted that if she was ever in trouble, she would be the first to turn up in a church. Sam saw it slightly differently:

> It's alright ... I like singing hymns and carols ... But if I'm at a service and there is a hymn, I have to look at other people to see if I'm keeping up with them ... or if I'm singing the right words in the right place ...

Sam had accepted his limitations at worship services. Nevertheless, as he had sung in the church choir as a boy, there is the suggestion that he would have been more involved if the services were more accessible. He explained his religious feeling:

> Yes, ... I believe in God, but I don't think he is continually working over everybody directing people's lives ... he let's you get on with it ... he's with you, but as a friend ...

Sam was not alone in seeing God as a friend. Anthony's wife Clare, also had a strong supportive sense of God. She said:

> Getting close to God ... gives [me] immense help and strength to cope with the problems [caused by having a deafened partner]. There are times when all ... [I have] to rely on is ... [my] faith, ... and that alone is enough to see ... me through many hard times.

Besides help coming from a person's faith, it also came from relationships formed with specific clergymen. Christine mentioned how her minister supported her through the loss of her hearing, her divorce, and the eventual death of her husband.

> my [Methodist] pastor ... [said to me] ... why don't you stop fighting with the evidence, [that I was losing my hearing], and start using it? So I went ... back to school and became a rehabilitation counsellor for deaf people and learned Sign ... '

In hindsight, Christine looked upon this time as a major mid-life crisis. Because of the support she received from her pastor and a rehabilitation counsellor, she was able to retrain and gradually moved into a career where she could use her experiences.

Lastly, Gwen recounted the importance of having a chaplain of the Deaf officiate at her marriage to Arthur:

> [Arthur and I] both Signed through the wedding. The chaplain ... Signed, and we employ[ed] a professional interpreter who ... interpreted all the service, ... and the chaplain did the hymns ... I had to learn [new] Signs as ... I didn't know the Sign for 'Holy' ...

The place of the chaplain of the Deaf, who in this case stepped in for Gwen's recently deceased minister, was crucial. He conveyed that Arthur and Gwen were not only making a commitment to each other, but also to the rights of Deaf people (Harris, 1995).

In reviewing this section on church involvement, there is a huge gap between what could be done for hearing impaired people and what is being done. Loop systems are a start, but many people are still missing out on what could be a more satisfying experience of worship.

Summary

This chapter has looked at the impact of hearing impairment on friendships, upon relationships with professionals, and upon religious involvement.

It emerged that the friendships of hearing impaired people could be improved immensely if revisioning took place towards the two primary adjustment processes required by hearing people to enable lip-reading: 'looking' and 'repeating'. For example, Noller (1984) points out that 'looking' is a positive interactive strategy in intimate relationships and helps to facilitate them regardless of hearing ability.

In a similar vein, Ree (1999), Stein (1935) and Tannen (1986) point to the immense value of 'repeating' both in Literature and as a basic human process. The revisioning of these two concepts could help to transform the caring obligatory aspect of communication with hearing impaired people to something of greater value and interest.

However, before looking and repeating can be processed, the ETTA factor must be acknowledged. It is about giving hearing impaired people access to general conversation in public as well as private places, to information, as well as to intimacy in specific friendships, in a similar way as providing a ramp for a wheel chair gives access to people with problems in mobility.

In the discussion of old and new friendships, it is clear that friendships do not necessarily diminish when one becomes hearing impaired. Much may depend on what social skills the person had before becoming deaf, and their proximity to old friends. Indeed friendships are and could be formed on the basis of reciprocity and equality. This was acceptable as long as it was understood there would be an instrumental aspect of the friendship from the beginning. It also emerged that two deafened people, Joy and Sam, found helpful understanding in cross gender relationships.

Overall hearing wives were more worried about their deaf husband's social network than the men themselves. These wives appeared ignorant of how men develop friendships. There was a suggestion that a feminine style network might be appropriate for a man especially during a time of 'adjustment'.

The analysis of hearing impaired people's relationships with professionals was seen in the context of social network formation where there is a disability, using Unger and Powell's three levels of intimacy (1980).

It is recognized that prelingually Deaf people, as represented by Arthur in this study, and well supported in the literature, have a long history of grievances with professionals especially with doctors, teachers and social workers, whom they feel are responsible for instilling feelings of inferiority in many prelingually deaf people. Clergymen, on the other hand, have managed to retain a helpful image.

Discussion concerning how doctors could better help their hearing impaired patients to accept their hearing aids indicate the benefit of doctors being more human and open in talking to their patients about hearing loss. Just because doctors cannot operate, does not mean that they have nothing to offer.

From examining the impact of hearing impairment on social networks, we will now explore its impact, specifically on elderly people, when a hearing partner has died leaving the hearing impaired partner to cope on their own.

CHAPTER 10

Bereavement

Introduction

In this chapter we examine the consequences of the ending of a marital relationship through the death of one partner when the bereaved partner also has an acquired hearing loss. Interesting though the experiences of younger people are, in practice, they form only a small proportion of the hearing impaired population. For example at least three-quarters of the 7.5 million adults with hearing loss in the UK are over 60 years old. In the 61–70 age group, at least a third have some degree of hearing loss and at least 10 per cent have a loss which is moderate or worse. In the 71–80 age group, over half have some degree of hearing loss and at least 20 per cent have a loss which is moderate or worse (RNID, 1990). Consequently an ever-growing older population means that hearing impairment will become an increasingly common, sweeping, and insidious condition in society, resulting in its developing significance and need for recognition as a social problem.

A comparative case study approach is used here to examine the adjustment of a widower, Max, and a widow, Theo. The interviews took place after they had both lost their respective spouses and had acquired a hearing loss. There were other losses present such as the loss of status which results from being an elderly person and retired, but this was seen as more peripheral to this analysis. Whereas widowhood has received a certain amount of scholarly attention (Marris, 1986; Parkes, 1987), with a few exceptions (Mouser *et al.*, 1985) the lives of widowers have been neglected. Another reason for focusing on a widower is that recent findings suggest that men are

closing the gap with women and dying later than in the past
(Church, 1995). In this study, 'access' was given by Max's two daughters and their families which made it possible to obtain a particularly
rich profile of him in his roles as father and grandfather. This makes
for a certain imbalance in this chapter as the widow, Theo, could not
offer her family for the study because her only son and his family
lived in the USA. However, an examination will be made of how she
created an adopted family and had a highly developed social
network.

The salient factors which made it possible for Max and Theo to
integrate their losses so that a new equilibrium could be established
will be analysed. Questions raised with reference to 'adjustment'
were about such factors as proximity of kin, proximity of friends,
personality and relational skills, past career experiences, the quality
of the previous marital relationship, the maintenance of personal
control, the proximity of 'community care' programmes (Hearing
News, 1992; Finch and Groves, 1980), lip-reading classes (Woods,
1986) and 'self-help' groups for hearing impaired people (SHHH,
1983:), specifically for elderly hearing impaired people who live
alone (SHHH, 1989).

There will also be a short exploration of the psychosocial unconscious healing processes used by Max and Theo which enabled them
to come to terms with the double loss of their respective spouses and
normal hearing. Lastly, the basically positive accounts which follow
are necessary to balance the largely negative literature on elderly
hearing impaired people (Gilhome-Herbst, 1983).

Marital breakdown

It is understood that a satisfactory marriage provides protection
against physical and mental ill-health because it acts as a buffer
against the effects of anxiety and stress (Dominian *et al.*, 1991).

However, a gender imbalance emerges in marital research
suggesting that such benefits for men far outweigh those for women
(Bernard, 1982). Consequently, when these strong emotional
ties between adults are broken, the severance is often accompanied
by anger, anxiety and depression, exacerbated if the break is

unexpected or undesired. The Holmes and Rahe's Social Readjust-ment Scale (1967) which measures life events through life change units, puts the death of a spouse at the top of its list while divorce and marital separation are also very high on the scale.

Thus marital breakdown, regardless of its exact cause, usually generates enormous amounts of stress over a long period of time. The family therapy and sociological literature explores how the family system responds to the death of a loved one (Walsh and McGoldrick, 1991; Bowen, 1991). Besides the impact on the welfare of the family as a whole, marital breakdown has an effect on the physical and emotional health of the individual adults (Marris, 1986) and children (Clulow and Vincent, 1987). Married people of both genders have been found to be emotionally and physically healthier than people who are not (Dominian et. al.,1991)

Marital breakdown as experienced in bereavement through the death of a partner

The finality of death is often portrayed as the closing off of relation-ship options, making it an emotionally overwhelming crisis for most families. Although the death of any family member carries with it a sense of grief, the death of an elderly person who has lived a full life does not usually arouse the degree of anger and sadness often associ-ated with untimely death, nor does it carry the potential for major gender role changes as it does when it occurs with young or middle-aged family members.

Sudden death of a significant family member throws the family into severe shock and sometimes 'emotional shock waves' occur. This network of 'after shocks' can occur anywhere in the family system (Bowen, 1991) in the months and years after the death. Even-tually the shock wears off and the bereavement process begins. The family is forced in due course to come to grips with stages of grief. Grief here is defined as the psychological process of adjustment to loss and involves feelings of numbness, pining and depression (Parkes, 1987). In most cases recovery is achieved and there is a reor-ganization of the family system and a reinvestment in other relation-ships and life pursuits (Walsh and McGoldrick, 1991).

Psychologically, individuals experience grief as an expression of a profound conflict between contradictory impulses. On the one hand, one needs to consolidate all that is still valuable and important in the past, and preserve it from further loss; and on the other, it is important to re-establish a satisfying pattern of relationships in the present where the loss is understood and accepted (Marris, 1986).

Determinants of the outcome of bereavement

Adjustment to the loss of a partner is initially worse for women, but more difficult for men in the long term. While attitudes are changing, husbands traditionally occupy a larger part of the life-space of their wives than the wives do of their husbands. For example, the wife's roles, plans and problems tend to be husband-centred and she may be reliant upon him for money, status, and company to a greater extent than he is on her. However, the literature also suggests that while overt manifestations of grief are more pronounced in women than in men, it is the women who are the first to recover from bereavement in the long term (Parkes and Weiss, 1983). In fact there is evidence that widowhood can be a liberating transition for women after which a flowering of new activity may follow involving new periods of parenting and step-parenting (Maas and Kuypers, 1974; Troll, 1971). For men also, new parenting experiences remain a possibility until the end of their lives.

While gender is undoubtedly a highly significant factor in determining the outcome of bereavement, other factors need to be considered. Briefly they may be divided into four categories: (a) background experiences of loss; (b) relationship with the deceased prior to death; (c) concurrent social factors of the bereaved partner for example, sex, age, personality, socio-economic status, religion, nationality; and (d) subsequent support, secondary stresses and life opportunities experienced after the partner's death (Parkes, 1987).

Elderly people who are hearing impaired are sometimes called in 'double jeopardy' (Becker, 1980). They normally suffer from presbycusis, a high frequency bilateral loss (Vernon et al., 1982).

We will now take a closer look at the lives of Max and Theo.

A comparative case study of bereavement: a widower and a widow

Because the elderly and disabled identities of Max and Theo were acquired over time, biographical details are of central importance in understanding their experiences (Cornwell and Gearing, 1989).

Max: description and background

Max was a tall, athletic-looking man who carried his 81 years with dignity. He had lived alone since his wife, Dora, had died seven and a half years earlier. He had been a teacher, headmaster of a secondary school in London, secretary of the borough's Teaching Association, and eventually president of the National Union of Teachers for one year. As we encountered in Chapter 7, Max had two adult daughters: a teacher and a social worker. The younger, Margaret and her family, lived in a house further up the hill in the street where Max lived; while the elder, Esther, lived further away, but in the same locality. This arrangement had made it easier for Dora to care for her grandchildren when their daughters went back to work. However, both daughters recalled that they had seen very little of their father while their mother was alive, as he was so involved in his teaching activities, a situation which they did not wish to repeat with their own children.

Thus almost by default, Max now in retirement, found himself able to keep in regular contact with his five grandchildren from the ages of 11 to 25. From his daughters' perspective, living close by made it easier to keep an eye on their father's welfare although this was often a difficult task due to ambivalence on both sides (Barry, 1995; Warnes, 1993).

Theo: description and background

Theo was a petite, slightly-stooped white-haired woman of 84. Behind a personable manner appeared to lurk shrewdness balanced by an enormous sense of fun. Like Max, Theo had formerly been a teacher. For the last seven years, she had been the headmistress of a primary school. Unlike Max who retired at 65, Theo was able to carry on until 71 because she worked in the private sector.

Theo felt that it had taken her three years to come to terms with her husband, Will's, death which had occurred four years prior to the interviews. He was ten years older than her and had been a pharmacist and an optician. They had one son, Philip, who was currently in the Head Office of a major oil company in Washington DC. Until four years ago, he, his wife and three children had lived nearby, so it was a double loss for them to leave the country just prior to his father's death. Although Theo's natural family no longer resided in England, she had many familial relationships (Gubrium and Holstein, 1990), a strong faith and rarely felt alone.

Remembering their partners

Max introduced discussions of his beloved wife, Dora, by saying how very beautiful she was, illustrating this by showing two photographs, one of her as a young girl, and one taken just before she died. His manner of doing this was like a ritual, an apparent effort to seek a sense of partial closure (Boss, 1991).

Max recalled:

> so I don't know how I [managed everything] ... if I hadn't had the wife I ... [had], I couldn't have done it ... because I was ... [rarely] at home some evenings, ... she was always here when I came back, looking after my daughters, ... the grandchildren, and also ... me ...

Max acknowledged his good fortune in having married such a devoted and nurturing woman, although Dora may have sacrificed something of herself so that both her husband and daughters could be high achievers. He gave a moving account of the day Dora died:

> She had a heart attack and was in hospital for a short time. She had come home and appeared to recover somewhat. It had been a beautiful summer's day. I suddenly realized about a half an hour before she died that she was dying. After it occurred, I went to my Roman Catholic neighbour and asked her to say a prayer even though I'm not a religious man. I felt a light had gone out of my life.

While Dora died relatively unexpectedly (Pittman, 1988), Theo recalled that Will's condition gradually deteriorated and it was necessary for them to move house and buy a bungalow which was accessible to Will's wheel chair:

> [Will] ... used to go ... in ... [his] wheelchair ... [on] a ramp, ... [so that] he could
> go right up to the edge of the patio ... In the spring there are daffodils ... all the
> way around ... [the house] it was nice to think that he was happy ... [here].

Will's eventual death at 89 appeared to leave his family free from any lingering guilt or grief and they could get on with their lives. Max, on the other hand, took longer to come to grips with his wife's death, perhaps partly because it was so unexpected (Walsh and McGoldrick, 1988).

Another partial explanation emerged in a discussion of friends. Max reflected:

> Well, the friend I had for life, I lost. Yes, that was my wife ... I don't think ... I
> have a mate [or colleague] outside the family [now]. I've had them in the past,
> but with the passing of the years, I haven't got them.

Max, like most men of his generation, undoubtedly cultivated context bound relationships which emphasized sociability (Allan, 1989). He also appeared to satisfy what needs he had for intimacy by relating to his wife and occasionally his family. Because seven years had passed since Dora's death, it was a little surprising that Max had not cultivated more 'special relationships' outside his family (Mansfield and Collard, 1988) where he could get back in touch with 'lost' aspects of himself, for example, young teachers with political interests.

Theo also cherished memories of her husband, Will, but they were of a different order from Max's as her marriage had contained some major disappointments and less emotional closeness. Thus Theo did not feel towards Will the same overflowing gratitude which dominated Max's account of his relationship with Dora. Theo speculated on the causes of their problems:

> [Will] was in World War I ... the strain on a young man as he was then, from 18
> years to 22 years, in the trenches must ... have made a difference to his outlook,
> to his personality and he said he was afraid, and I had always to cope with that
> ... He had the Military Cross and Bar in the war ... so he was very good, but it
> left him [very nervous] ... for no reason at all ...

Theo saw Will's lack of sexual desire for her as directly connected
with his war experiences which is likely to be partially true (Kaplan,
1979). They did manage to consummate their marriage while on
holiday 14 years after they were married. She recalled:

> I was very patient ... you didn't think of skipping off because you were disap-
> pointed, ... we went to Devonshire for a holiday [and conceived our son, Philip]
> ... The problem with Will wasn't so obvious after having a child. I suppose in a
> way, [becoming a father] put him right ...

Despite these regrets, Theo had pleasant memories of Will. She was
particularly proud of his fine mind and speech which she could hear
long after she had acquired her hearing loss, as well as his achievements in founding a nursing home for pharmacists. She recalled one
favourite memory twice:

> my husband ... was [ill] in bed, ... and I remember [going] into the bedroom
> very quietly [when] I [thought] he was asleep, .. and he suddenly said some-
> thing to me, ... and I said, 'Oh, I'm sorry, I hoped ... you wouldn't hear', ... and
> he said, 'No I couldn't hear you, but I could sense your spirit in the room' ... I
> thought that was so sweet ... it was nice ...

Thus she and Will had been able to transcend the disappointments
in their marriage, leaving a deep affection at the time of Will's death.
Referring to their earlier difficulties she said:

> I'm glad that [I] did have patience, because it was worth it, and I think today
> some people don't wait to see if somebody's worth it.

Perhaps Theo's optimistic nature and faith were one reason why she
was able to have the necessary patience. Max, on the other hand,
appeared to have more difficulty with his own company. This could
be a more general gender factor (Parkes, 1987) as we shall see in the
next section.

Being there for bereaved parents: a special son and daughter

Max recalled how his younger daughter supported him:

> my daughter ... pops in most evenings, if only for a few minutes ... she realizes
> it's a lonely life, especially when it gets dark at half past four, and you've got to
> wait until ten o'clock before you go to bed ...

Margaret understood her father's need for companionship. Her ability to be a confidante provided a buffer against some of the negative effects of retirement and being a widower (Lowenthal and Haven, 1968). She reflected:

> sometimes I don't feel like going, ... to some extent it's a duty, but I do also enjoy his company ... Since my mother died, I think I'm closer to him than I've ever been in my life ...

While both daughters felt genuine compassion for their father, they were uncertain about how much care was appropriate. While it was not possible to talk with Theo's son, Philip, his involvement with his mother was revealed in some of her stories. She recalled:

> Philip had to go [to the USA] on the 2nd of March and Will died on the 18th ... it was a difficult time for me ... Philip ... had only just taken up his new position, ... he came back straight away ... and stayed a week ... made all the arrangements and helped me ...

Philip put his mother's welfare first despite the demands of his new job. Theo was especially moved by Philip's helpfulness in rearranging her sleeping area. She remembered:

> Philip was so sensible ... he moved my bed into the main guest room, and [gave me his father's] saying 'You will like this ... a firm bed not so soft as your old one ... we'll put your bed into the other room' which we did, and so I ... have ... that nice firm bed that belonged to [Will] ever since.

Philip's action in moving his father's bed into his mother's room, besides being a practical gesture, could also be interpreted as a symbolic gesture by which authority as head of the family was transferred to his mother. It also helped Theo to identify with her husband and thus to integrate his loss (Pincus, 1974).

Although Philip was with his mother during times of transition, what was missing in her life was the more traditional day to day 'tending' family care which took place in Max's family to a certain extent (Bulmer, 1987).

While Max was most appreciative of the care he received, for example, his daughters' provision of a daily evening meal, this scenario also had its frustrations in that he often felt a burden (Montgomery et al., 1985).

The discussion will now shift to examine Max and Theo's social network.

Social networks: family and friends

While many of Max's affective needs were met by his daughters' families, his lack of peer contacts appeared to result in his feeling a low sense of psychosocial well-being (Roberto and Scott, 1986). Hearing losses in elderly people may make them feel they lack credibility as friends (Beattie, 1981) as the communication difficulties caused by the loss can take away the feeling of 'equality' that is such a basic concept of most friendships (Nussbaum *et al.*, 1989).

Max appeared to partly compensate for this by attending the Crawley Hard of Hearing Group. Margaret recalled:

> [my father] was very lonely when my mother first died, ... and that [is maybe] what prompted him to go ... I [didn't think he would like it]. He's not that sort of person really ... He goes along every Friday afternoon and he really enjoys it ...

Attendance at self-help groups has long been a coping device for people with a disability (Ainlay *et al.*, 1986). Max obviously understood the value of group support, perhaps because of his long involvement with the teachers' union. He explained:

> [the local Hard of Hearing Group] is a little get-together and I like it, perhaps because I'm meeting people with my own affliction, we have ... a disability in common ... it's purely social ... nothing remedial, ... and I like the people there, ... and I go to support them.

People with disabilities are often helped to find the strength to 'accept' their disability through social acceptance and approval by other disabled people (Fishman, 1959). Generally, perceived similarity is associated with liking. There is also the suggestion in Max's account that 'shared stress' leads to enhanced cohesion (Schachter, 1959).

While Max enjoyed the atmosphere of the group as a whole, Theo, a co-member and friend, had a special relationship with its coordinator, Edith. Edith saw to it that Theo had all the assistive hearing devices she needed, and generally ensured that she did not get too isolated, for example by inviting her to church services with refreshments at her house afterwards. On the other hand, if very occasionally illness threatened, it was Theo's neighbour, Edie, who did errands for her such as fetching medicine from the pharmacy.

While Theo relied on her neighbour, Max relied on his daughter. Margaret recalled how she 'interpreted' for her father at the surgery:

> If [my father sees] Dr Benson, ... [who] speaks very quietly, ... [he] can't hear half of what he says, ... so usually I go along and act as an interpreter ... Because I feel under pressure, ... I'm working full time, ... I want to make sure that I get him well. I'm not always confident that he will give the doctor the full story, ... it's me being in control, that's what it's all about.

Margaret acknowledged her mixed motivations in her treatment of her father. On the other hand, she discriminated and did not accompany him to his pernicious anaemia clinic. There were other situations where Max's desire to keep his independence and his daughters' desire to be caring caused some irritating situations. Max's elder daughter, Esther, related such an incident:

> [Before he went] to London for the evening ... I said, 'You're 80 and there're some "rough toughs" around, and you shouldn't be out on your own at night ... I do worry about you.' He ... [told me when] he was going to be home, ... [and then] he didn't come ... We [rang] and [rang] to check he'd come in, like a mother with her child really ... Finally ... he rang ... ten past 12 o'clock ... [My sister] duly went down to Crawley [in the car] to pick him up. He [told her], 'I've waited 40 minutes for the bus, [but] it didn't come.' She said, 'Why didn't you call when you got off the train?' ... 'Oh, I didn't want to trouble you,' he'd said and she replied 'Why didn't you get a taxi if you didn't want to trouble us?' and he replied, 'Oh, I didn't want to spend the money.' Now that's the sort of person he is ... he's annoying trying to be independent ...

Esther's attempt to reverse roles with her father (Ungerson, 1987) was not effective. While exasperating to his daughters, Max's fight to maintain his control and autonomy was another factor essential to his sense of well-being (Doyle and Gough, 1986). Thus Theo and Max were forced by fortuitous circumstances to reverse what might be traditionally expected.

While Max found himself surrounded by a protective natural family, Theo found herself in the midst of an adopted family consisting of neighbours, friends, professionals, tutees and a cat. It emerged that this reversal had its advantages and disadvantages. While Max had to fight to keep himself from being over protected, Theo was rarely allowed the physical 'tending' traditionally given to women in their eighties (Bulmer, 1987).

We will now explore how Max and Theo coped with memories of the past and their lives in the present.

Memories of past successes and reinvestment in the present: social network continued

While Max had found a new equilibrium in his life, he, nevertheless, missed the enormous enjoyment he had experienced in living the active part of his life. He recalled:

> I enjoyed my life as a teacher. I enjoyed my family life, there were lots of ups and downs you know, feelings of despair, feelings of elation, of triumph and joy, and it's all a lovely old mixture like a currant cake.

Max could not only remember functioning normally, but functioning well under considerable pressure:

> At Easter I go to a conference of the National Union of Teachers. I was President twenty years ago and my hearing was perfect ... I mean I was in the chair at a conference of 2,000 delegates ... every day for a week, and anybody in the back row who asked a question, I could hear. But if I go to that conference ... today, [I'm] ... still eligible to go as a trustee, I can't hear if I'm [sitting] behind the microphone.

In the manner that he was able to 'let go' and integrate the loss of his wife, Max was able to mourn and integrate the loss of his career (Mattinson, 1988), and accompanying perfect hearing. He managed to do this as demonstrated in his willingness to learn how to cook and clean. At the same time, he maintained a certain minimal involvement in the politics of the teaching profession, in community activities, the neighbourhood, sports activities, and he kept himself in a relatively healthy state. This had included getting himself one hearing aid from the National Health Service, and enrolling in a lip-reading class.

While Theo also felt diminished by the loss of her husband, job and hearing, she appeared a little more resilient than Max. She recalled:

> I enjoyed [my work] so much ... I used to write a lot ... and the very first article I had [published] was in *The Lady*, an article called, 'My Lovely Job', because that was how I felt about it ...

Theo acknowledged great good fortune in her job, family, general health and ability to make a rich variety of friends. She explained:

> I will always have friends anywhere, even say if I were to move to the USA to be nearer my son, ... I have no intention of sitting in a corner ...

Although much more confident than Max in her capacity for making new friends, she was equally very appreciative of her very old friends. She remembered:

> the friend for life in mind, ... Margo, I met her when I was teaching, ... she was Scottish and very much better-educated than I was, ... she was a good friend because she thought I could do anything ... About five years ago, ... she went blind ... and now her greatest pleasure is talking to me on the telephone one, two, three times a week. [It's supportive for me too] because when I finish, I say, 'thank you'.

Another member of Theo's network was her hearing impaired younger sister, Jess, with whom she spent Christmas every year. Theo reflected:

> if anybody is deaf, ... they get ... into the way of hearing you the second time ... I get a bit tired of saying everything twice, ... in the same sort of voice, ... [it seems] in a way [that they] are not attending, ... but that's unkind because [Jess] can't help it.

While the two sisters had different degrees of loss, Max and Theo had relatively similar degrees of loss, but heard different frequencies. In other words, Theo heard the birds singing while Max heard the lower piano notes.

Hearing loss is sometimes considered to be less of a problem for elderly people since the statistics suggest it is to be expected (Humphrey *et al.*, 1981). It was, therefore, of specific interest to investigate the response to diagnosis and onset.

The onset of hearing loss

Max first noticed his deafness not long after his wife died. He recalled:

> I lost my wife ... in June 1982 ... [then] my hearing was perfect, but ... perhaps a year ... [later], I began to go deaf ... and I've often wondered whether the shock of bereavement,.. [her death] was [so] unexpected, was a contributory cause ...

Both daughters had heard a different story. Margaret remembered:

> Well I think we were aware of ... [father's deafness] when my mother was alive
> ... because she always used to say 'Oh, he's so deaf!' ... I think probably towards
> the end of her life, she used to get a bit frustrated ... [about it].

It was, therefore, likely that Max's hearing had begun to deteriorate
before Dora died. Bereavement has been known to trigger the first
appearance of chronic conditions in family members resulting from
'emotional shock waves' (Bowen, 1991). The truth may be twofold in
that it is possible that Max's deafness began before his wife's death, but
was accelerated afterwards. Perhaps Dora had protected Max from
the knowledge that he was hearing impaired because she had automatically accommodated to his need for repetition. Moreover, her
death exposed him not only to his own deafness, but also to his other
dependency needs, such as being unable to cook or clean the house.

Theo was more sophisticated than Max about hearing loss
because her mother and sister were hearing impaired. Her gender
may also have helped her to face reality more quickly (Doyle and
Paludi, 1991). Theo recalled how she first became aware of her
problem at 70 while teaching:

> As soon as I found that I wasn't able to hear the little children, ... I remember
> asking a friend, ... 'I think I'm getting deaf, what should I do?' And she said,
> 'Well I think you should do something about it' [and] I got a hearing aid.

While the onset of hearing loss occurred to Max and Theo in very
different ways, the next section reveals their shared sense of loss
when confronted with what they could no longer fully enjoy.

Loss and difference

Max discussed how it was for him on the telephone:

> [With] friends, ... I say 'go slower and speak clearly', [sometimes other] people
> speak very quickly and then I lose it.... I have to put up with it ...

He recalled what it was like with music and drama:

> I can hear music better than I can hear speech, ... but if there's a play, a drama,
> a lot of it I miss and, if you miss parts of a drama, you may miss the vital lines
> and it's ruined, so I don't waste my time listening to plays ...

Telephone conversations and television were no longer as pleasurable for Max as they once had been. Theo also had a frustrating time with the phone especially when she volunteered her services to the local RELATE association and wasn't able to respond appropriately to distraught clients.

Nevertheless, she felt she managed some fairly successful conversations with her grandchildren in the USA because she had an amplifier on her home phone and they knew how to speak to her. Theo had similar feelings to Max about the television, but her feelings of loss in relation to music appeared to be specifically connected to her piano:

> The piano I ... thought ... [to] sell, ... because I don't like to play it now my husband's gone, ... [sometimes] it doesn't sound right, ... and then I go on, and it ... becomes right.

The piano, like her new bed, was another link with Theo's husband, and she was very concerned to do the right thing about it. It appeared that decision-making and the autonomy involved became a strain for her sometimes. Again Max had the opposite problem in that he longed for more autonomy. His grandson, Greg, highlighted how Max's hearing loss could cause mild embarrassment at the family dinner table:

> If I say something like, ... 'Can I have an extra tin of peas for lunch?' ... my grandad will think it's something [important] and start saying, 'What did you say?'

As we have seen, meal times with Max and his family were sometimes difficult as family members were uncertain how they could proceed normally, and at the same time be sensitive to their grandfather's feelings of exclusion.

Margaret was right when she said that her father was more comfortable in his own home. There he was able to maintain control and decide what was and was not important 'to hear' (Kyle, Jones and Wood, 1985). This in turn was likely to facilitate his hearing in that conversations directed towards him were easier to hear than those across him.

While Theo did not regularly interact with her own grandchildren, she helped small children with reading. She explained:

> I've got a little Asian boy who comes here on Thursday ... I can [not] understand what he's saying, but I can guess ... [I] ... teach ... [him] to read ... [with]

flash cards – I [say], 'Put out all the ones you know and then tell me.' Then I can hear him ...

Theo's confidence in her ability to communicate with small children meant that she could sustain her teaching role despite her hearing loss and the little boy's heavy Asian accent. Theo and Max both reported very little difficulty understanding their own grandchildren as will be described in the next section.

More from and about grandchildren

Max did not feel that his hearing impairment in any way obstructed his relationship with his five grandchildren. He related:

> Oh I sometimes say to [my younger grandchildren], 'you must go a bit slower'. 'Alright grandad, we'll try again' so they're very cooperative ... No I don't think [being deaf] has damaged my relationship with [my grandchildren] at all ... they're very loving children ... they come and see me just as they would before I was deaf ...

All the grandchildren had made an effort to relate to their grandfather and he with them with considerable success. In fact Max was able to develop a relationship with each grandchild around common interests, mutual support, or involving tasks which needed doing. While he had difficulty in the family group, Max's experience of life meant that he had acquired an excellent ability to manage intimacy with his grandchildren when they visited him individually.

One of Max's five grandchildren, 13-year-old Greg, had acquired a unique perspective of his grandfather's bereavement. He recalled his enjoyment of being with him:

> I reckon I've got a bit closer to grandad ... since my grandma died. I was quite close to her [too] ... Now I go down on my own in the evening[s] ... and we get on quite well ... We just sort of sit ... if I crack a joke, he gets it ... He understands what I mean ... I'll laugh with him, and I ... won't let him get away with anything and he never lets me get away with anything.

He had observed changes in his grandfather's behaviour:

> He sort of looks after us now ... before I got to the stage when I could ... go out on my own, ... [he would] look after us, and we['d] stay the night, and we always had boiled eggs and soldiers in the morning ... But when grandma died,

he didn't cook for himself [or anyone else], he didn't really know how to, ... he just sat there ...

As part of the acceptance and integration of Dora's death, Max had identified with her and become more nurturing (Pincus, 1974). This also meant that 'help' was still reciprocal. Margaret explained:

my dad helped me out considerably at different times ... When the children were a bit younger, ... he would always have them if they were ill and I couldn't take the time off, ... he would always do other bits of shopping for me locally if I asked him to. It's a bit of a two way thing really, I know that I can rely on him.

Margaret's comments reflected the 'intergenerational solidarity' which Dora had built in to familial relationships (Bengston and Cutler, 1976). Greg added:

I think in his own way, he does like his own company ... Sometimes we go down there, but ... you get the sort of feeling that he's glad when you go as he wants to be quiet, and when you're leaving and there's a good TV programme on that he likes, you sort of say goodbye to him and [he replies] 'bye bye' [and] I sort of laugh inside [when this happens]. I know what he likes.

Max's intense manner in watching these programmes was different from other hearing impaired grandfathers in this book. For the latter, there was a fascination with a world they had never experienced; for Max it had been a world that he had experienced, if only for a relatively short time. For both, television served as a link object and compensation (Becker, 1980).

Greg and Max had developed a unique form of intimacy which a grandfather and grandson could develop when they were similar in temperament, see each other daily, and share marginal adult status (Cunningham-Burley, 1987; Hockey and James, 1993).

Theo knew that she had not been as fortunate as Max as her grandchildren had been out of the country. But she was, nevertheless, grateful for what was given:

[My grandchildren] have been back every year since they went away, and I don't have any difficulty hearing them, ... well apart from saying 'speak up a little louder: I can't hear your quiet voice' ... Yes, [occasionally I have to ask them to repeat] ...

Theo, like Max, could be direct about her need for clear speech from her grandchildren. She described how letters also helped:

> When Philip writes [his weekly] letter [to me], I can see what the children are doing in the house, what Richard is doing in the garden ... the rabbit got out and did something funny – I'm really there with them, and it's wonderful ...

Theo's deep understanding of children generally helped her to fill in the missing blanks in her grandchildren's lives. On the other hand, she was delighted when one actually came for a visit. She related:

> I didn't know Diana so well until she stayed with me, and ... she has the 'organization' ... When she came from Heathrow, she would come to Victoria, ... ring me up to say that the train was just leaving Victoria, but she had already booked her coach to Leeds the next day, ... she is just how I like ...

While Theo missed observing the development of her grandchildren first hand, communication flowed across the Atlantic and she was well informed. Her hearing loss had not been an obstacle in this process because of the family's great facility for writing letters.

Summary

In this chapter, a case study approach was used to focus on the lives of a widow and widower. Both had lost their partners within the last ten years and both had an acquired hearing loss. It emerged that the widower had more difficulty adjusting to bereavement than the widow. This is supported in the literature in that despite men's larger investment outside the home, they nevertheless, often have a deep and enduring relationship with their spouses.

It was necessary for both Max and Theo to experience certain psychosocial processes throughout their bereavements so that they could refocus on their lives, for example, their need to 'accept' their losses with the accompanying sense of 'stigma', 'to identify' with the positive characteristics of their dead partners and 'to integrate' the past reality with the present.

While Max denied he was coping well, no doubt because he felt so diminished without his wife's support, he made an exceptional adjustment to the circumstances in which he suddenly found himself. Max was helped by the fact that the families of his two daughters lived locally providing support, he had acquired excellent relational skills so that he could relate closely to his family, and he was basically happy with his life choices. The latter meant he could take further risks, for example, his joining of the local Hard of Hearing Group.

Theo also made an excellent adjustment to her bereavement. As her husband had been an invalid for many years, she was more prepared than Max had been. However, the actual death of her husband was deeply felt as they had managed to transcend disappointments which had occurred earlier in the marriage. Theo was like Max in that they were both outgoing and thoughtful people who had acquired excellent relational skills. These in turn helped them through their times of loss.

Theo differed from Max in that her 'little bit' of family lived in the USA. This was not to suggest that she was emotionally isolated from them since visits, letters, and telephone calls were exchanged. As it emerged, Theo was in fact very important to her son's family both as its inspirational 'head', and as a 'half way house' between the USA and the UK. What was missing for her was a more traditional 'tending' of physical needs which took place in Max's family, along with the rich relationships which he was able to nurture daily with some of his grandchildren. Theo and Max were thus forced by fortuitous circumstances to reverse what might be traditionally expected. For example, when their respective spouses died, Max found himself surrounded by a protective natural family. Theo, on the other hand, found herself in the midst of an adopted family consisting of neighbours, friends, former colleagues, professionals, tutees and a cat. It emerged that this reversal had its advantages and disadvantages. It meant that Max had to sometimes fight for his autonomy, while Theo seemed occasionally overwhelmed by hers.

The focus of this chapter has been on the complete breakdown of the marital relationship through death and the aftermath of bereavement. The next chapter will explore some social policy issues involved with rehabilitation for people with hearing loss.

PART III

Social Policy Issues and Conclusions

Chapter 11

Provision for People with Acquired Hearing Loss: How Adequate in the UK?

Introduction

In the process of carrying out the research for this book, an investigation was made into services for hearing impaired people in the UK, especially services provided by the NHS. These services target people who have lost some degree of hearing, from mild to total, after they have acquired speech rather than a condition apparent at birth. While RNID statistics (1996) suggest that 17 per cent of the population are deaf and hearing impaired, there are in fact 150 people who have acquired hearing loss for every one person who is born deaf. We are, therefore, discussing rehabilitation in the traditional sense and not services for people who are prelingually deaf which are covered by social and educational provision and the voluntary sector.

The World Health Organisation in 1958 stated that 'rehabilitation' was not only about restoring the disabled person to his previous physical condition, but was also about developing fully their physical and mental functions'.

The dominance of the 'medical model' at this time led to this definition being accepted by social policy and disability scholars, although ideas began to change in the 1970s (Townsend, 1979; Sainsbury, 1970). The 'medical model' places considerable emphasis on assessing the individuals' objective performance audiologically and in terms of their ability to communicate (Alpiner, 1980). However, this model has been highly contested by scholars in the disability (Oliver, 1983) and deaf fields (Padden and Humphries, 1988) because it sees the problems that disabled people experience as being the result of their disability. When professionals follow this model, they interpret their task as helping individuals to adjust to their disabling condition. This is experienced by disabled people as a form of reductionism and is usually accompanied by lowering self-esteem and confidence. Eventually disabled people are expected to resocialize themselves among 'their own' (Goffman, 1963).

Oliver and his colleagues (Swain *et al.*, 1994) argue that the problem does *not* lie within the individual as the 'medical model' of rehabilitation suggests, but within society at large. In this 'social model' of disability, the problem is removed from the individual and placed in the environment. In the specific case of hearing impaired people, the 'social model' removes the problem from afflicted individuals and focuses on their right of access to spoken English. Oliver and his colleagues find fault specifically with the medical/rehabilitation model due to its focus on the issues of 'normality' (Morris, 1994) and 'dependence' (Oliver and Barnes, 1994), which are seen by them to be social constructions. Nevertheless, Oliver does accept the need for a period of rehabilitation.

Both the medical/individual model and the social model have valid points, and so there is much to commend a *both and* position which draws from each model when appropriate. The discussion now shifts to a clarification of terms.

Adjustment and reconfiguration

Jones, Kyle and Wood prefer to speak of 'adjustment' to the acquisition of hearing loss and define it as:

> [the] change in [the patient's] behaviour, belief, relations, or interaction occurring in the period from the onset of hearing loss whenever that actually is (1987: 54).

This term was adopted in reaction to earlier research where rehabilitation models took their place within a psychiatric framework (Kraepelin, 1915). This apparent obsession with psycho-morbidity studies continued as in the work of Markides (1983) and Thomas and Herbst 1980). However, the latter did acknowledge that while their research helped to quantify psychological disturbance, there remains no satisfactory explanation for what it was about hearing loss which made those afflicted so vulnerable to mental illness. Gradually researchers began to investigate this question with varying results (von der Leith, 1972). Of particular interest are the findings of the Bristol team. They conclude that the degree to which an individual can tolerate the reduced and varying access to information at home, socially and at work will determine the degree of 'adjustment' (Wood, 1993).

While the term 'adjustment' is a more restrained term than 'rehabilitation', it nevertheless is seen to be unsatisfactory by Oliver (1983) and other sociologists and social administrators. They argue that it is also socially constructed and comes from bereavement theory making the assumption that some aspect of the person with a disability has died or is unwell (Sleeboom-van Raaij, 1993). They feel that this is a simplistic perspective which does not take in the full and diverse experience of individual disabled people (Campling, 1981). In other words, some disabled people may actually be very healthy and/or have never felt much grief since they have never known life without their disability (Lenny, 1994).

Yet, despite its limitations, the term 'adjustment' accurately describes the process experienced by the majority of people in this study who became hearing impaired. This process of 'adjustment' was experienced before, or simultaneously with, getting on with their lives. Another term suggested by scholars is 'reconfiguration' (Padden, 1989). This word focuses on the 'matter of fact' linear nature of a multi-dimensional reshuffle in all processes connected with communication. This reshuffle takes place simultaneously with the gradual awareness of family (Wood, 1993) and friends that there is a hearing impaired member in their midst requiring ETTA (Effort, Time, Thought and Attention). As I have suggested, the ETTA factor is about having the energy required to help a hearing impaired person take their rightful place in both formal and informal conversations.

Although behaviour change inevitably occurs long before a formal diagnosis is made, it is at the time of diagnosis that people begin to meet professional rehabilitators and the adjustment phases begin. In the UK, this is mainly a time of hearing aid provision rather than the intervention of support services. This is not to say that hearing aid provision does not reduce the problem for some people or that surgery and medical treatment are not occasionally sufficient. Rather, it is that middle-class English norms dictate that people with problems should live as best they can. Although there are signs that this attitude is changing (Kent County Social Service, 1995–6), people with hearing impairment are at present inclined to forego any professional help that is in fact rightfully and helpfully theirs (Corker, 1994).

While this discussion is relevant for our understanding of traditional rehabilitation methods, this chapter focuses specifically on the young profession of Hearing Therapy. As the study progressed, the importance of the specific role and boundaries of Hearing Therapists emerged suggesting the need for analysis and policy formulation. This emergence is in conjunction with a more general discussion currently taking place between other rehabilitation professionals, namely Audiological technicians, Audiological Scientists and Deaf Workers.

First we analyse the present situation of the profession of Hearing Therapists, and the historical and political context from which it has developed. Current services will be compared with the more developed services offered in some other European countries. After discussing policy recommendations, the focus will shift to the help given by informal rehabilitators: spouses, significant others, and by the person's own initiative.

Hearing therapy in the UK: a brief synopsis

We must begin by asking what the initial consequences were of the DHSS's decision to substitute experience and lip-readability for a graduate degree for those seeking entry into the profession of Hearing Therapy (DHSS-ACSHIP, 1975). First, the multi-faceted nature of acquired hearing loss which strikes at the very heart of human communications was ignored (Jones, Kyle and Wood, 1987). With the medical model still in ascendant at this crucial time of formation, the nature of acquired hearing loss was reduced to the physical process of not hearing. Secondly, although some individual Hearing Therapists are graduates and beyond, the training specifically required to date is only for one year beyond secondary education. This requirement, while giving the profession a certain platform from which to launch itself, has also along with underfunding, significantly limited Hearing Therapists in their work. However, at the time of writing, a concentrated effort is being made to develop the training and raise standards within the Department of Health (Greenaway, 2000) and within the Hearing Therapy profession itself as will be discussed.

I argue that if Hearing Therapists are to be truly effective, they must receive a much more rigorous training specifically in counselling theory and practice along with more opportunities for self-development and evaluation than they currently receive.

This is in addition to a certain amount of medical/audiological training which they presently receive. This would help Hearing Therapists to facilitate the 'therapeutic alliance' (Beck, 1991), to understand the systems approach and to use the three family dimensions: adaptability, cohesion and a facilitating communication (Olson *et al.*, 1983). It is in the forging of this alliance that a truer 'adjustment' may be obtained.

Before discussing these concepts further, we will focus on how the idea of Hearing Therapy was conceived.

Hearing therapy's historical context: The ACSHIP Report

The Provision of the Chronically Sick and Disabled Person's Act (1970) highlighted the appalling gap in services for people with acquired hearing loss. This was further confirmed by the Rawson Report (1973). In September 1974, a subcommittee of the Department of Health and Social Security's Advisory Committee on Services for the Hearing Impaired People was asked to consider the rehabilitation needs of adult hearing impaired people. The brief given was to make recommendations specifically in reference to the role of the NHS.

The subcommittee elected to concentrate on the core of the rehabilitation process which was the follow-up of patients attending ENT departments. They agreed that it was not sufficient simply to fit a hearing aid and to assume all recipients would automatically and spontaneously acquire a skill in its use. Previous surveys of users of the old Medresco box hearing aids had found as many as 39 per cent did not use the hearing aid every day, and that 10 per cent did not use their aid at all. This suggests that the lack of follow-up rehabilitation services for patients with sensorineural deafness had frequently resulted in severe disappointment, and further sad waste of individual abilities and public money (DHSS-ACSHIP, 1975).

The published report of the sub-committee called for the creation of a class of experienced workers with special training in the skills required. The report detailed the roles, skills, training, personal attributes, qualifications, prospective salary range etc., which would be required by the new worker. The Hearing Therapists' role was seen to be to assess the extent of the disability and to formulate a rehabilitation strategy. The aim was to raise the patients' communication performance to the maximum possible and to maintain it at this level. This was seen as a very complex process because of the multiplicity of factors involved namely how much and what kind of residual hearing the patient had, how much innate lip-reading ability was possessed, what was their communication lifestyle, what were their social needs, and what was their general motivation to make the adjustments involved. It was further suggested that the assessment would be designed to elicit the patient's own definition of their communication problems; for example, what did the patients regard as difficult situations, and in what circumstances did they arise? (Hegarty et al., 1983).

Recommendations made in the body of the report and diagrams found in the Appendix suggest that the new profession of hearing therapy was to be seen as one member of a multi-disciplinary patient care team consisting of a student in audiology, a technician, a teacher of the Deaf, and a Speech Therapist. They all, in turn, were responsible to the ENT consultant concerned. It was also acknowledged that part of the rehabilitation process might be provided by people from other disciplines outside the ENT department, namely psychiatrists, psychologists, Health Visitors, disablement resettlement officers and family and social counsellors (see Appendix C). Furthermore, the special problems and needs of hearing impaired people might involve discussions with family members, neighbours, employers, teachers etc.

In evaluating the response of the Department of Health and Social Security to these recommendations, it is important to understand that 1975 was possibly the worst time to publish them. By 1976, as a result of the oil crisis, economic and political ideas had turned a somersault, as social service expenditure which had been increasing since the end of World War II, became severely checked because of the lack of hope in improving overall economic growth. Some attempt was made, however, to implement the ACSHIP report as the following section will explain.

Health Circular (78)11: the birth of Hearing Therapy

In 1978, the Department of Health and Social Security considered ACSHIP's recommendations and issued Health Circular (78)11 (DHSS-Circular HC (78)11, 1978). It announced the establishment of a new NHS profession called 'Hearing Therapists' The most pronounced change from the original recommendations was the qualifications required of the profession. While the ACSHIP report had clearly recommended that training for hearing therapy began at the graduate level, Health Circular (78)11 read:

> The post will be suitable for mature candidates with at least two years experience, preferably in the NHS or with a local authority social services department, in working with the deaf or hard of hearing. While no specific academic qualifications are laid down, the course is an intensive one year course of professional training at higher education standard and is primarily intended to add to previous training and experience in working with Deaf people. An ability to speak clearly and to be lip-readable is essential.

Earlier in the circular it was also noted that, 'a majority of the population (in the UK) would not satisfy such a requirement' (DHSS-Circular HC(78)11, 1978)

While the substitution of experience and lip-readability for a graduate degree was an astute practical and financial decision, it was in fact immensely short-sighted. Without rigorous training leading to a degree and beyond, Hearing Therapy lacks an intellectual foundation on which to build and develop. This has consequently led to a narrowing of the service and provoked widespread controversy within the profession as well as without.

In adopting this position, the DHSS appears to have lost sight of the multi-faceted nature of hearing impairment. It is not just about the physical process of not hearing, nor is it about the frustration experienced in losing information and social control. It strikes at the very heart of all human communication. Seen from this perspective, the problem is much deeper and more encompassing in that the ability to hear is a primary component in all relational processes especially those within the family. Here we come full circle as many observers see the well-functioning family as a cornerstone of participative citizenship.

Much recent research and professional experience suggests that there are more helpful approaches to facilitating the adjustment of hearing impaired people. Before discussing them, it is important to look at some of the strengths of the service which Hearing Therapists are currently providing in the UK as well as examining what is available in the USA.

Contemporary Hearing Therapy

As is understandable with a young and developing profession, the emphasis of the training and the work are continually changing. To be able to form an accurate and up to date picture, there is a need for much more thorough on going research than has yet been undertaken (Hegarty *et al.*, 1983). The Hearing Therapy Service, like other NHS services, varies from one part of the country to another in its focus and strengths. However, some generalizations may be made. Hearing Therapists are mostly based within a hospital or community health setting. They may act as a link between the patient and the rest of the Team responsible for treatment which now includes the ENT Consultant, Audiological Scientist and Audiological Technician. Hearing Therapists specifically focus on help with hearing aids, lip-reading instruction, auditory training, advice about environmental aids, tinnitus management and counselling individuals and their families. Nicholls (1992) describes this latter service with individuals as the process of exploring the patient's own feelings about what has happened to them which hopefully enables them to adjust to the loss as much as possible. She updated these remarks (2000) by adding with regard to Hearing

Therapy training: 'There is, and has always been, a great stress on working with the family and during the social effects of deafness blocks, we develop this theme.'

Publications of the British Society of Hearing Therapists and the job description given to particular Hearing Therapists show that Hearing Therapists aim to provide a very comprehensive service which has broadened since the early days of its inception. By February 1998, there were just over 100 Hearing Therapists working in Britain. There are believed to be some 5 million people with acquired hearing loss, 25 decibels or more. To develop an adequate provision, there is a desperate need for more Hearing Therapists.

While most Hearing Therapists have broad based roles, some specialize in particular areas, for example, in balance rehabilitation, cochlear implants, people with learning disabilities, and support before and after operations. The work can also include the provision of information and training to voluntary organizations and other professions, as well as information to the general public (BSHT Career Leaflet, NDG). While trainees during their one year receive 38 counselling sessions each of three hours' duration, along with supervised experience in the field, the majority of their training remains more technical and practically based. In 1992 the Centre for Deaf and Speech Therapy (The City Literary Society) tried out a new approach in that they introduced the National Vocational Qualification whereby students take more responsibility for their own learning (Levene, 1992). While this might improve the quality of training, it in fact does nothing to remedy the fundamental difficulties inherent in Hearing Therapy training which are just beginning to be addressed at various levels. Firstly, Dr Peter Greenaway, Chief Scientific Officer in the Department of Health, is considering the establishment and consolidation of what he hopes will be an all-graduate Audiology profession within the NHS. He hopes to establish basic training which will be acceptable to all three groups: Audiological Scientists, Audiological Technicians and Hearing Therapists and that this will be in place by 2001/02. He believes that all three groups have current difficulties with career development, education development and motivation which lead towards the larger problem of professional self identification (2000). He is also

concerned that at the moment there is no registration programme
for Hearing Therapists nor is there a consistent or robust educational programme. He has recently established a Forum composed
of representatives from the three groups in an effort to discuss what
some of the issues are in the development of a registration policy and
a more cohesive knowledge base.

There is also one new initiative that has developed within the
Hearing Therapy profession itself. The University of Bristol now
offers a Diploma in Hearing Therapy for professionals in related
Audiological fields who wish to strengthen their work in Rehabilitation Audiology (Nicholls, 2000). On top of this, a working party has
been formed for the purposes of establishing a MSc in Rehabilitation Audiology. Short professional courses in Deafness and Rehabilitation are also on offer in 2000/01 at the Burwalls conference
Centre in Bristol.

Britain is not alone in entering the field of Hearing Therapy
relatively late. Professional counselling help in the USA for people
with acquired hearing loss has been 'hit or miss'. Training for counsellors with specific expertise in the difficulties caused by an
acquired hearing loss is just beginning to be recognized as a need
(Sloss Luey, 1992) and the necessary training provided as illustrated
in the Federally operated Certification in Rehabilitation Counselling programme in the USA (Commission, 2000) Within this
programme, it is then possible to specialize in work with both deaf
and hard of hearing persons as illustrated in the course provided at
San Francisco State University (Nemon, 1998). Success here is
partly the result of awareness programmes sponsored by two
national consumer organizations: Self Help for Hard of Hearing
People and Association for Late Deafened Adults. Despite the
progress, the majority of people providing human services of all
kinds are not knowledgeable about how to adapt communication
for people with hearing loss and are completely unacquainted with
the psychosocial issues and experiences of those populations (Sloss
Luey, 2000).

Before looking at other countries in more detail, it is appropriate
to explore the concept of rehabilitation counselling specifically
counselling designed to be of use to people with acquired hearing
loss.

Rehabilitation counselling for people with acquired hearing loss in the UK

The experience of both clinicians (Harvey, 1989) and researchers (Oyer and Paolucci, 1970) and the evidence produced in the study indicates that a hearing impairment is often disturbing and stressful to intimate family relationships. Family Therapists, in their use of the systems approach, frequently point out that when objects of a system are actually people in relationship with other people, one of the most important attributes of that system is communication behaviour (Galvin and Brommel, 1991).This is further confirmed by findings that a disability or illness, especially one involving a barrier to good communication with one member of the family, is likely to have a profound effect on the family as a whole (Oyer and Oyer, 1985). Conversely, the attitudes of family members can have a strong influence on the overall adjustment of the unwell members (Jones, Kyle, and Wood, 1987).

If counselling had been part of the general rehabilitation programmes available to families in the study, an attempt would have been made by the counsellor to build a 'therapeutic alliance' with them. This is done by showing empathy towards the couple along with professional competence in dealing with the problems they present. This approach would have facilitated a more accurate picture of their difficulties. While an understanding of the medical/audiological problems and issues is certainly valuable for families, the findings in my study suggest that it is an understanding of the psychosocial ones which lead couples/families to forming deeper bonds with an enriched perspective. For example, hearing impaired parents in this study who found appropriate ways to discuss openly the true nature of their hearing impairment with their children, were much closer in a healthy way to them than parents who hid, joked, blustered or treated it as a taboo subject.

When members of a family present themselves for counselling, the counsellor attempts to engage everyone in the therapeutic alliance. As a feeling of trust develops, the counsellor may look with the family at the role of one member's hearing loss within the family system. How does each member of the family feel about it? Can they be honest about their negative feelings, and can they go on to discover positive ways of coping? Some of the issues explored could be concerns about autonomy, intimacy, sense of loss and stress. The study's findings suggest that these are specific topics which are deeply felt, but are often difficult to discuss. Perhaps most crucial, the clinician must have the skill to help the family discriminate between those concerns which result directly from the hearing loss and those concerns which have resulted from other factors. For example, the four couples in this study who divorced were at first likely to blame the hearing loss of one partner for the breakdown of their relationship. After further investigation, it was revealed that there were, in fact, many factors involved with the hearing loss being *one* exacerbating factor. It is also important for the clinician to have an awareness of the importance of the family dimensions arising from the three dimensions of family life: cohesion, adaptability and a facilitating communication (Olson *et al.*, 1983), along with many other psychosocial concepts which a thorough grounding in counselling theory and practice could provide. Such courses are currently available at many universities. Of particular interest are a MSc course at the University of Bristol in Counselling in Primary Care/Health Settings (Etherington, 2000) and a MSc course at the University of Brunel entitled Counselling in Health Care and Rehabilitation (Griffiths, 2000).

Now that we have briefly examined the current state of Hearing Therapy in the UK, and briefly explored the concept of rehabilitation counselling in the context of people with acquired hearing loss, it is appropriate to examine what is happening in other countries. As Sweden is the country which probably has the most evolved approach in this field, we will focus on it in greater detail.

Sweden:a holistic approach

The members of the original ACSHIP subcommittee did not see their recommendations as innovative. As a team from the Department of Health and Social Security had visited the Scandinavian countries in 1973 in order to obtain information about their services for hearing impaired people, the ACSHIP subcommittee was aware that considerable progress had already been made there, especially Sweden and Denmark. For a comparison with the British system, it is instructive to look in some detail at the Swedish programme for hearing impaired people. In Sweden, there is an extensive programme of local auditory services which provide assistance to people with acquired loss. Besides this, there is a National Labour Employability Institute based in Uppsala with special resources for disabled people specifically for those with acquired hearing impairment (Lundmark and Hellstrom, 1989). It is financed by the Swedish Government and the programme offers hearing rehabilitation combined with vocational rehabilitation and employment counselling. The activities of the Institute aim to eliminate recurrent difficulties and prepare for problems in employment primarily in the regular labour market.

When a hearing impaired person arrives at the Institute, they are asked to spend three days talking to several professional experts who assess them from different perspectives. As this is done, a treatment plan is developed with concern for the whole person. A Hearing Therapist will check the person's hearing aid. It will be exchanged for a new one if it is not appropriate. The Speech Therapist will examine speech production and speech reading. If there are other physical problems such as tinnitus, a medical audiologist will discuss ways in which this might be helped. If the hearing impaired person suffers from stress and tension, the physiotherapist may help with relaxation exercises.

As there is a strong understanding of the psychosocial consequences of hearing impairment, the person will meet a social adviser and a psychologist. This is often followed by the person's family arriving for a 'Family Day'. At this time it is hoped that family members will deepen their knowledge and understanding of some of the problems which the person has to face. The person is often asked to write down their own expectations of themselves. If they feel they fall short in some way, the psychologist may offer some supporting short term psychotherapy. If the person has progressed this far, they will then be encouraged to take part in employment counselling discussions with a small group of other hearing impaired persons. Once the person establishes the kind of job they would like, counsellors work with the local labour exchange so that appropriate training and eventual job placement takes place. When this has occurred, the hearing impaired person is discharged from the Hearing/Employability Institute, and may receive further counselling and support at the local level.

While every rehabilitation programme has its limitations, the Swedish programme, which offers both intensive and long term help, has a high rate of success in returning hearing impaired people to their homes and new jobs with improved functioning and confidence (Lundmark and Hellstrom, 1989). This suggests definite advantages in the holistic approach when a person has a hearing impairment. It is important to clarify that in focusing on Sweden, it is not being suggested that the UK is entirely without holistic treatment centres for hearing impaired persons. The rare places where such treatment does exist are either registered charities with very specific goals such as the Link Centre in Eastbourne, or experimental collaborative programmes with regional health authorities and social services such as the Birmingham Centre for Deafened People. Neither programme has the secure government backing which may be found in some European countries.

Given the cultural and historical differences in the development of Continental European welfare states, particularly the frequency with which their benefits are conditionally linked to labour market participation, it is unlikely that Britain will go fully down the Swedish road in the near future. Currently, Sweden is undergoing a programme of privatization designed to cut costs and to increase the choices of recipients of social service provision. How exactly this will affect services to those who are hearing impaired remains to be seen (Martin, 1992). Nevertheless, we can learn from the contrasts in service provision found in the two countries. There are questions about the use of time and money, the training and use of professional personnel, and the profile of hearing impaired people more generally. Among the many questions which could be explored, two particularly stand out. First, why is it that a Hearing Therapist in the UK may be given one year of training with an undefined theoretical foundation after secondary education before becoming qualified, while therapists working with hearing impaired people in Sweden, Denmark, Holland and Germany, are required to attend a much longer period of training?

Here it is helpful to make a more precise comparison with the 'Hearing Pedagogues' of Denmark. Pedagogues must all be qualified teachers (four year college training and/or university education) with an additional 14 months specialized training in the education of hard of hearing children. The Swedish have a similar requirement for their Hearing Therapists. Most Hearing Therapists have an education as a teacher for about two years. After a certain period of time teaching, they may add a special training (diploma) learning specific details about hearing impairment. Three terms of further study are required for working with hearing impaired people and four terms for working with deaf people.

Secondly, why is it that a hearing impaired person in Sweden is encouraged to talk to a team of six to eight professionals while in the UK, a person with the same problem is considered fortunate to encounter one dedicated, but overworked Hearing Therapist? So far in Britain, to date, only a little over 100 Hearing Therapists have been trained out of the 300 originally recommended (Attwell and Watts, 1987).

Whatever the response to these questions, evidence for the need to develop and/or reform the current system in the UK is clear.

A way forward

While it is hopeful and exciting to see various initiatives which are currently afoot on behalf of the profession of Hearing Therapy, it is important simultaneously not to lose sight of the historical development of the profession and the very real difficulties which have attended its development. Attwell and Watts (1987), Hearing Therapists themselves, with great honesty identified a number of difficult areas. First, responses to a questionnaire sent to members of the Hearing Therapy profession revealed that the majority of them felt that the Department of Health and Social Security were at fault in their Health Circular (78)11 in choosing to ignore the original ACSHIP recommendations, and for finally suggesting that the entry requirements for hearing therapy training should be 'candidates with no specific academic qualifications'. It is believed that such free entry has no doubt contributed to the poor career and salary structure; and this in turn undermines the Hearing Therapists' ability to meet fellow therapy professionals on an equal footing. Secondly, there are fundamental concerns among Hearing Therapists themselves about aspects of the training course, namely the general status and length of the course, entry requirements etc., especially compared with other professionals using the name therapist (for example, Occupational therapy offers a three year programme, Speech therapy has a three or four year programme) (Hegarty *et al.*, 1983). Thirdly, the present economic climate and NHS changes have meant that many hospitals are stripping themselves of all but essential services. Because Hearing Therapy is relatively new and unestablished, it is unlikely to be given priority. Yet the case is otherwise in some other European countries, for example Germany (Fromberg, 1989), Holland (Hooglander-Mensink, 1992), Denmark and Sweden (Lundmark and Hellstrom, 1989). This is not to suggest that British hearing therapists lack international recognition (Levene *et al.*, 1996).

A second way forward, as we have seen in Chapter 8, is to teach awareness that a communication problem belonging to one member of the partnership or family in effect belongs to the whole kin network. If the responsibility of rehabilitation becomes a challenge for both the couple and the family, the negative aspects of the disability (for example irritability when unable to hear) have a much greater chance of being transformed. In this respect. there is much to learn from the Swedish system with their 'family days'. It is possible that that family involvement will no longer be seen as a mere option in rehabilitation work, but as an early and fundamental requirement. This is supported by the Bristol researchers when they say:

> the resources available to hearing therapists have been totally inadequate. Hearing people are participants in hearing loss and need to be involved overtly in the adjustment process. Their involvement should occur as soon as hearing loss is suspected. (Jones, Kyle and Wood, 1987: 224)

Thirdly, every effort should be made to recruit hearing impaired people as Hearing Therapists. As research suggests (Ridgeway, 1991), equal status of interviewer and interviewee is likely to facilitate a more honest and helpful exchange of information thereby leading to a better provision of service. There are other factors, however, besides status alone operating in a user/provider relationship. This suggests that whether deaf or hearing, hearing therapists require good supervision if staff development is to occur (Mattinson, 1977).

Undoubtedly, if Hearing Therapists and other related professionals became more united in their understanding of the importance of the problems of people with acquired hearing loss, a stronger joint effort could be made to consolidate their resources, experiences and skills. With the additional support, Hearing Therapists would be in the position to expand their own existence, improve training, status, career structure, professional knowledge and methods. The eventual outcome of all these improvements would be the establishment of an adequate rehabilitation service for the ten million people with acquired hearing loss in the UK.

Dr Peter Greenaway's initiative towards an all-graduate Audiology profession appears to be going in the right general direction. At the same time, MSc degrees in counselling, rehabilitation and audiology have/are being developed at a number of universities which will make it possible for motivated Hearing Therapy graduates to develop to a much higher standing than is currently possible.

The systems perspective, although not without fault, for example, in that it does not sufficiently address gender issues (Wheeler *et al.*, 1991), seems to offer one of the most promising theoretical frameworks for Hearing Therapists to use. The purpose behind this strategy is to encourage the collaboration of the family in the rehabilitation process or a 'household therapeutic alliance' which could expand to become a 'household/family friendship therapeutic alliance' so that obligations and enjoyment, duty and choice, may ideally be contained together within household, marital and family boundaries, revitalized over time.

Two explicit social policy issues arise from this discussion. First, what is the best institutional framework in which to provide adequate rehabilitation services: hospitals, in the community care programme, or in other institutes or centres as found in Scandinavia? Secondly, with the introduction of the quasi-market to the NHS, and the provision of many services by the private sector, how should the services be best coordinated?

If it is the case that some of the formal rehabilitators are not doing as effective a job as they might, how are rehabilitation/reconfiguration processes being managed? Let us now consider the experiences of people interviewed in this respect.

Informal rehabilitators

Study participants often mentioned professionals who were not formal rehabilitators; for example help was given by a psychotherapist, a psychiatrist, a Speech Therapist, a homeopathic doctor, a singing teacher, a marital therapist, a head teacher, and a Methodist minister. Most of these people operated in hearing settings, and could be seen to overlap with the first level of social support (Unger and Powell, 1980) discussed in Chapter 8. While the literature (Kazak and Marvin, 1984) argues that it is the informal rather than the formal social support networks which are the most crucial to families where there is a disability, this study suggests that the situation is far more complex. It appeared that the boundaries between formal and informal care had merged in certain families. Four out of the 16 hearing impaired people in the study had married a spouse in a rehabilitation related profession. For example, Barbara had married Ben, a lawyer interested in disability issues; Joe had married Sarah, a lip-reading teacher; Henry had married Kay, a teacher of English as a foreign language; and Arthur had married Gwen, an infant teacher who knew BSL and hoped to become a teacher of deaf children. Another seven people in the study had married 'wise others' (Goffman, 1963) in that they were people who were already aware of strategies for managing stigma and loss. They had sufficient internal and external resources to cope without resentment with the extra emotional demands of having a hearing impaired spouse.

The question may be asked how it was that a quarter of the hearing impaired people in the study married partners in the rehabilitation field? Such marriages certainly assured a certain 'place' for deafness within the boundaries of the marriage. Conversely, the hearing impaired spouse could give a certain credibility to the career of the rehabilitation professional. Moreover, the rehabilitation specialist would 'know' about the problems without its implications having to be articulated. This ideally would save energy, time and embarrassment for the hearing impaired spouse.

Yet again, the reality observed in these relationships was more complex. With some couples, there was danger of emotional overload for the rehabilitation professional when being 'at home' was too much like being 'at work'. Considerable objectivity had to be maintained so that the boundaries between the two spheres were clear. Lastly, additional stress could be felt by the helping professional because of the self-imposed high expectations of always being 'the expert' (Corker, 1994).

The focus shifts to more self-help forms of rehabilitation.

Reconfiguration; significant others and self-help

Ideally the goal of medical and psychosocial rehabilitation is for the responsibility of its administration to be taken over by the patients themselves and in this way, except for the occasional check-up, outgrow their patient role (von der Leith, 1993). A common feature of most of the people interviewed was their willingness and ingenuity in doing this. Some took up old interests with slight alterations, while others discovered new activities. The most noticeable characteristic of these activities was the enormous variety and range they represented. The three most commonly mentioned interests were going on foreign holidays, religion and the development of a deep faith, and watching television. Not surprisingly, all three activities have a strong visual component. Other more individual interests included operating Hornby trains, astrology, leading a sign language choir, meteorology, being a remedial reading teacher, viewing art exhibitions, DIY, economics, self sufficiency, the Labour Party and reading. Even music and taking up a foreign language were mentioned.

Socialization with other hearing impaired people appears to be one factor in promoting psychological health. Thirteen out of the 16 hearing impaired people interviewed in the study had contact with other hearing impaired people through sign language classes, self-help groups, or as hearing impaired deaf/charity administrators. However, this contact ranged considerably from being very superficial to a deep commitment, perhaps a reflection of the acknowledged ambivalent attitude of stigmatized members of society to 'their own' (Goffman, 1963).

Generally it may be concluded that rehabilitation/reconfiguration processes are continuing, long lasting and few generalizations can be made about what particular individuals ought to do in order to become well 'adjusted' as hearing impaired people. It is partly because of this individualistic nature of the process which makes appropriate counselling so necessary.

Summary

The focus of this chapter is on the formal rehabilitation services currently offered to hearing impaired people in the UK, specifically viewed within their historical/political context. The young profession of Hearing Therapy is discussed with its roles and boundaries. Hearing Therapy's particularly vulnerable situation resulted from the decision in Health Circular (78)11 to disregard the DHSS's subcommittee's recommendations. The consequence of this downskilling of Hearing Therapy has been a tendency to undertake rehabilitation in too limited a context, ignoring the multi-faceted nature of hearing loss and the need to engage in a holistic way with many aspects of life. At this point in time, an attempt is being made by Dr Peter Greenaway, Chief Scientific Officer of the Department of Health, to reverse this process by considering the establishment of an all-graduate Audiological profession. He hopes that it may be launched by 2001/02. MSc Degrees in counselling and in rehabilitatiion have also been established which may be taken if Hearing Therapists wish to develop their skills further.

It is believed that the primary task of a well trained Hearing Therapist is to facilitate the formation of a 'household/family friendship therapeutic alliance' by effectively using an understanding of the systems approach and the three family dimensions: cohesion, adaptability and a facilitating communication, as well as other helpful and appropriate psychosocial concepts.

This is because this study suggested that psychosocial concepts were as important if not more important than medical/audiological ones.

We now draw the threads of the book together in the two concluding chapters. The penultimate chapter will analyse the psychosocial perceptions of ' deafness as a difference' constructed by the study participants. Some charts have been devised to help us see how the different constructions and perceptions relate to each other. The final chapter will explore nine important themes which have emerged from the research.

CHAPTER 12

An overview

Introduction

We now develop an overview of the psychosocial constructions of all the relationships in this book in an effort to discover which factors were most crucial in facilitating more positive or negative constructions and perceptions of 'deafness as a difference'.

To provide a context for this overview, it is helpful to recall the study's working hypothesis which is that couples who contain a hearing impairment within their marriages need to assess how it is affecting the quality of couple and family relational processes. If this is not done on some sort of regular basis as the family develops throughout the life-cycle/course, it is likely that these processes will deteriorate or not develop appropriately. This hypothesis was very general and dependent on the degree of hearing impairment and the age of onset.

While the literature argues that marriage/partnerships between hearing and hearing impaired people are rarely mutually satisfying, and therefore more likely to deteriorate, it emerged that such marriages were in fact 'good enough' if a certain 'quality factor' develops despite and/or because of a mild to profound hearing loss within the relationship.

Consequently, although adjustment to acquired hearing loss is associated with the time of onset and the degree of loss, as we have seen throughout, psychosocial factors, specifically those found in intimate relationships, may in fact be as important, if not more important, than medical factors in predicting long-term adjustment. This is because couples who have an unconscious 'couple fit', are able to psychosocially construct reality together. In other words, they develop a 'shared perception' of the way the hearing loss functions within their relationship. This shared perception focuses on their 'differences' as part of an anthropological/cultural model, rather than on illness or maladjustment as found in a medical model.

Chart of Spousal Shared Perceptions (SSP)

The highly personal perceptions of the 11 couples in the study were put on a chart of Spousal Shared Perceptions (SSP) (see Figure 12.1). The purpose of the chart is threefold: first to classify into groups the shared perceptions of 'deafness as a difference' and to see what characteristics each group has in common. Secondly, to assess whether the hearing loss is perceived as a major or minor factor in lifestyle, plans and goals of the couple. Lastly, to determine what factors within the couple's lives bring about a change in the couple's shared perception of 'deafness as a difference'. It is then hoped that this analysis will provide more effective insights for counselling intervention.

The plus factor

Along the positive to negative axis, four groups emerged. The first group was made up of two couples who had psychosocially constructed the meaning of 'deafness as a difference' so that it was seen positively or 'the plus factor' (PF). For example Arthur and Gwen had the shared perception that Arthur's loss was 'respectable and OK'; while Anthony and Clare saw Anthony's deafness as 'a blessing although sometimes problematic'.

The question was then asked what Arthur and Gwen and Anthony and Clare have in common, which would indicate why they were able to perceive 'deafness as a difference' in such positive terms?

Medically, Arthur and Anthony appear to have had opposite experiences with Arthur, congenitally deaf, and growing up in a deaf family; and Anthony, from a Nigerian family, deafened suddenly at age 31.

LABEL	PF PLUS FACTOR +	IF INDIFFERENT FACTOR		MF MINUS FACTOR –	FCF FAMILY CRISIS FACTOR	TOTAL NUMBER
SHARED PERCEPTIONS OF 'DEAFNESS AS A DIFFERENCE' IN MARRIAGE/PARTNERSHIPS OF PEOPLE STUDIED	1 RESPECTABLE AND OK 2 A BLESSING BUT SOMETIMES PROBLEMATIC	3 A STRESS FACTOR 4 A NUISANCE	5 AN INSIGNIFICANT FACTOR 6 A FRUSTRATION 7 AN OCCASIONAL SOURCE OF SADNESS	8 A PROBLEM TO BE WATCHED 9 A COMMUNICATION PROBLEM 10 A CHALLENGING PROBLEM	11 A SHARED BURDEN	11
CHARACTERISTICS						
LEVEL OF DENIAL	LOW	LOW	MEDIUM	LOW	LOW	
LEVEL OF ACCEPTANCE	HIGH	HIGH	MEDIUM	MEDIUM	HIGH	
LEVEL OF INTEGRATION	HIGH	HIGH	MEDIUM	MEDIUM	HIGH	
KIN NETWORKS	VERY SUPPORTIVE	MIXED SUPPORT	MIXED SUPPORT	MIXED SUPPORT	MIXED SUPPORT	
FRIENDSHIP NETWORKS	VERY ACTIVE	VERY ACTIVE	LESS ACTIVE	VERY ACTIVE	VERY ACTIVE	
PARTICIPATION IN SELF HELP GROUPS	ACTIVE	LESS ACTIVE	LESS ACTIVE	ACTIVE	ACTIVE	
THE HEARING PARTNER'S ATTITUDE TOWARD 'CARE'	EASY GOING	EASY GOING	EASY GOING	EASY GOING	EASY GOING	
NATURE OF LOSS PERSONALLY FELT BY DEAFENED PARTNER	AUTONOMY	NONE	BEING NORMAL	BEING NORMAL	AUTONOMY AND INTIMACY	
HOPE FOR THE FUTURE	HIGH	MEDIUM	MEDIUM	MEDIUM	MEDIUM	

Figure 12.1. Spousal Shared Perceptions

DEGREE OF HEARING LOSS	PF PLUS FACTOR + (1 RESPECTABLE AND OK; 2 A BLESSING BUT SOMETIMES PROBLEMATIC)	IF INDIFFERENT FACTOR (3 A STRESS FACTOR; 4 A NUISANCE)	IF (5 AN INSIGNIFICANT FACTOR; 6 A FRUSTRATION; 7 AN OCCASIONAL SOURCE OF SADNESS)	MF MINUS FACTOR – (8 A PROBLEM TO BE WATCHED; 9 A COMMUNICATION PROBLEM; 10 A CHALLENGING PROBLEM)	FCF FAMILY CRISIS FACTOR (11 A SHARED BURDEN)	TOTAL NUMBER 11
PROFOUND/TOTAL						
Joy					✓	
Sam						
Arthur	✓	✓				
Anthony	✓					
SEVERE						
Barbara			✓			
Joe				✓		
Henry			✓			
Robert				✓		
MILD/MODERATE						
Anne				✓		
Frank			✓			
Rachel		✓				

Figure 12.2. Degree of hearing loss related to spousal shared perceptions of impact of hearing loss on their relationship

TIME OF ONSET OF HEARING LOSS	AGE	LABEL: SHARED PERCEPTIONS OF 'DEAFNESS AS A DIFFERENCE' IN MARRIAGE/PARTNERSHIPS OF PEOPLE STUDIED	PF PLUS FACTOR + : 1 RESPECTABLE AND OK, 2 A BLESSING BUT SOMETIMES PROBLEMATIC	'IF INDIFFERENT FACTOR: 3 A STRESS FACTOR, 4 A NUISANCE	'IF: 5 AN INSIGNIFICANT FACTOR, 6 A FRUSTRATION, 7 AN OCCASIONAL SOURCE OF SADNESS	MF MINUS FACTOR – : 8 A PROBLEM TO BE WATCHED, 9 A COMMUNICATION PROBLEM, 10 A CHALLENGING PROBLEM	FCF FAMILY CRISIS FACTOR: 11 A SHARED BURDEN	TOTAL NUMBER: 11
BEFORE EDUCATION								
Barbara	Birth				✓			
Henry	Birth				✓			
Arthur	Birth		✓					
Joy	Infancy					✓		
AFTER BASIC EDUCATION								
Sam	18			✓				
Rachel	26			✓				
Anthony	31		✓					
Joe	37						✓	
Anne	38					✓		
AFTER MAJOR LIFE CHOICES MADE								
Frank	56				✓			
Robert	58					✓		

Figure 12.3. Time of onset of hearing loss related to spousal shared perceptions of impact of hearing loss on their relationship

ROLES OF HEARING PARTNER ON BEHALF OF HEARING IMPAIRED PARTNER	INTERPRETER	ADVOCATOR	EDITOR	PROMOTER	MEDIATOR	BUFFER
Mike (H) & Joy (P)	✓	✓		✓		✓
Julia (H) & Sam (P)	✓		✓	✓		
Ben (H) & Barbara (S)	✓	✓		✓		✓
Sarah (H) & Joe (S)	✓	✓		✓	✓	
Kay (H) & Henry (S)	✓		✓	✓		
Gwen (H) & Arthur (P)	✓	✓		✓		
Adam (H) & Anne (M)	✓			✓		
Simone (H) & Frank (M)	✓					
Mary (H) & Robert (S)	✓					✓
Richard (H) & Rachel (M)	✓				✓	✓
Clare (H) & Anthony (P)	✓				✓	

H = Hearing
P = Profound/total deafness
S = Severe hearing loss
M = Mild/moderate hearing loss

Figure 12.4. Communication roles of hearing partner

PRACTICAL ROLES OF HEARING IMPAIRED PARTNER IN MARITAL RELATIONSHIP	DOMESTIC HELP	BREADWINNING (PAY)			PARENTING	GRAND-PARENTING	SPOUSAL SUPPORT	CULTURALLY INTERESTING
		Higher than partner	Same as partner	Lower than partner	Primary Parent	Supportive Parent		
Joy (HI) & Mike (H)	✓			✓	✓		✓	6–7
Julia (H) & Sam (HI)	✓	✓			No Children		✓	7–8
Barbara (HI) & Ben (H)	✓		Volunteer		✓		✓	8–9
Sarah (H) & Joe (HI)	✓		✓		No Children		✓	7–8
Kay (H) & Henry (HI)	✓		Student			✓	✓	7–8
Gwen (H) & Arthur (HI)			Student			✓	✓	9–10
Adam (H) & Anne (HI)	✓			✓	✓		✓	7–8
Simone (H) & Frank (HI)	✓	✓				✓	✓	9–10
Anthony (HI) & Clare (H)	✓		✓			✓	✓	9–10
Robert (HI) & Mary (H)	✓		Volunteer			✓	✓	9–10

H = Hearing
HI = Hearing Impaired
Culturally interesting (Scale 1–10)

Figure 12.5. Practical roles of hearing impaired partner

ONSET OF HEARING LOSS IN RELATION TO THE TIME OF PARTNERSHIP ACKNOWLEDGEMENT	PF PLUS FACTOR + 1 RESPECTABLE AND OK 2 A BLESSING BUT SOMETIMES PROBLEMATIC	IF INDIFFERENT FACTOR 3 A STRESS FACTOR 4 A NUISANCE 5 A COMPLAINT 6 A SIGN OF OLD AGE	IF INDIFFERENT FACTOR 7 AN INSIGNIFICANT FACTOR 8 A FRUSTRATION 9 AN OCCASIONAL SOURCE OF SADNESS	MF MINUS FACTOR – 10 A PROBLEM TO BE WATCHED 11 A COMMUNICATION PROBLEM 12 A CHALLENGING PROBLEM	FCF FAMILY CRISIS FACTOR 14 A SHARED BURDEN 15 AN UNSHARED BURDEN 16 AN INTOLERABLE BURDEN	TOTAL NUMBER 16
BEFORE ACKNOWLEDGEMENT						
Gwen & Arthur	✓					
Julia & Sam		✓				
Sarah & Joe						
Kay & Henry			✓			
Barbara & Ben			✓			
Grace & George*					✓	
AFTER ACKNOWLEDGEMENT						
Joy & Mike					✓	
Simone & Frank			✓			
Rachel & Richard		✓				
Mary & Robert				✓		
Anne & Adam				✓		
Clare & Anthony	✓					
Dora & Max*		✓				
Theo & Will*		✓				
Kay & Fred*				✓		
Christine & Jack*					✓	

* Reconstructed relationships before the breakdown of intimacy.

Figure 12.6. Time of onset of hearing loss related to spousal shared perceptions at the time of partnership acknowledgement

From a psychosocial perspective, however, these two couples have many similarities. For example, the 'quality factor' is found in the relationships of both couples. Specifically, both the hearing impaired and hearing partners have succeeded to a certain degree in integrating 'deafness as a difference' within the boundaries of their marriages. None of the four individuals involved needed to make use of the psychological defence of 'denial' which meant that true acceptance and compassion could develop.

Secondly, from an anthropological/sociological perspective, both couples understand how to manage oppression and 'outsider status' constructively. In practical terms, this meant that Arthur and Gwen and Anthony and Clare already had initial social networks and self-help groups in place which more or less accepted both the deafness, and the deaf and hearing partner as a couple. Thus both couples were protected from the socially constructed negative attitudes of the dominant hearing culture towards people who are deaf, as well as negative attitudes towards couples where one partner is an 'outsider'. Because these two couples felt a certain security with themselves as a couple, they could get on with their lives immediately despite the difficulties they experienced.

Indifferent factor

Five couples were classified as belonging to the next group where the meaning of 'deafness as a difference' was perceived by the couples as an indifferent factor (IF). IF was broken down into two subgroups on the basis of how well the hearing impairment was emotionally integrated in to the marriage and/or whether the 'quality factor' was present. Deeper analysis revealed that Sam and Julia and Rachel and Richard, who had perceived 'deafness as a difference' in their relationships to mean 'a stress factor' and 'a nuisance' respectively, had fully integrated the hearing loss and its implications into their relationships. The fact that Sam was profoundly deaf and Rachel had a mild/moderate loss did not appear to be factors which influenced the couple's shared perception and the integration process. A certain degree of acceptance and compassion was needed in all cases.

The second subgroup was composed of Henry and Kay, Barbara and Ben, and Frank and Simone who had perceived 'deafness as a

difference' to mean respectively 'an insignificant factor', 'a frustration', and 'an occasional source of sadness'. While these partners
talked openly about 'deafness as a difference' within their relationship, it was observed that a collusion process took place. The hearing
spouses, for whatever reason, experienced the hearing loss as too
negative to be fully integrated into their marriages. Consequently,
many of the implications of deafness such as the need for extra
emotional support and understanding, were pushed outside the
marriage boundaries. For example, Barbara was an executive of a
Deaf charity and Henry was training to be a chaplain of the Deaf;
but rarely could either bring the daily difficulties of their situation for
acceptance by their families. This added to their personal isolation
and meant that their hearing family members lacked the enhanced
perspective of seeing their hearing impaired family members as
being both similar to and different from themselves.

Evidence suggests that difficulties in integrating 'deafness as a
difference' are more likely to appear when one of the partners has
late onset hearing loss, when they have married late, or when their
social networks are underdeveloped. In these cases, it appears that
there are insufficient amounts of what researchers claim to be essential for optimally functioning families, that is 'adaptability, cohesion
and a facilitating communication'. It is specifically these family
dimensions which encourage integration and are therefore part of
the 'quality factor'.

Minus factor

A 'minus factor' (MF) is represented by the third group which
emerges on the chart of Shared Spousal Perceptions (SSP). It
contains Anne and Adam, Sarah and Joe, and Mary and Robert
who psychosocially constructed the meaning of 'deafness as a difference' to mean respectively 'a problem to be watched', 'a communication problem', and 'a challenging problem'.

This group is distinctive because the hearing partners are more
consciously aware than in other groups of their strong caring function within their partnerships. This function was articulated by
Sarah and conceptualized in this study as ETTA, the Effort, Time,
Thought and Attention required by the hearing partner when

communicating with their hearing impaired spouse (specific roles undertaken may be found in Figure 12.4). Although ETTA was operating implicitly with other couples, there was less consciousness of it. There was also some shifting towards and away from this group. For example, although Anthony and Clare claimed Anthony's deafness was a positive factor, its problems were emerging daily. While Julia and Sam saw Sam's hearing loss as one 'stress factor' in their lives resulting in an indifferent factor classification, there remained the possibility that it would become more problematic if they were to have children. The latter example suggests that family transitions of any kind are likely to make couples revise their shared perception of 'deafness as a difference', and that it is likely to shift down the axis until a new equilibrium is found.

In acknowledging the validity of the ETTA factor, it needs to be seen alongside the knowledge that the couples' relationships are on the whole interdependent.

Family crisis factor

The last grouping to emerge is sudden deafness experienced as a family crisis factor (FCF). Mike and Joy perceived the meaning of 'deafness as a difference' in their relationship to be 'a shared burden'.

The question was then asked in what ways were Mike and Joy different from other couples so that their psychosocial construction was more negative? It was certainly not their basic relationship as they were a particularly well-suited couple, enjoying each other's company in both work and leisure. After deafness struck Joy twelve years into their marriage, they continued to maintain their shared perspective because Joy was an excellent lip reader and Mike was a natural communicator. Mike, as rated by the researcher, was a 'high adjustment' husband in that he not only allowed Joy's deafness to be fully integrated into the marriage so that the 'quality factor' was present, but he also took an interest in the intellectual and technical aspects of her condition. Two other deafened women in the study, now divorced, were not so fortunate.

While Joy kept her husband by her side together with a number of devoted friends, her sudden deafness meant that she had experienced a number of crucial losses. These were her loss of social autonomy, capacity for intimacy with her only son, of status and feelings of marginalization in that she was no longer her husband's business partner. These specific losses tainted what was given and lowered her enjoyment of life, resulting in the more negative joint perception of 'deafness as a difference'.

Summary of findings from the SSP chart (Figure 12.1) with accompanying Figures 12.2–12.6

The purpose of devising Figure 12.1 (SSP) is to investigate how perceptions of the meaning of 'deafness as a difference' in 11 couples compared with one another. Some general and some specific conclusions are made.

It emerges that five couples considered that 'deafness as a difference' had not made a major impact on their lives together. This is the indifferent factor (IF). The remaining six couples felt that 'deafness as a difference' had made a major impact on their lives and they form the plus factor (PF), the minus factor (MF) and the family crisis factor (FCF).

These highly personal psychosocially constructed meanings appear on the whole unrelated to the time of onset and the degree of loss (see Figures 12.2 and 12.3). However, they may relate to whether the deafness was present at the time of couple acknowledgement as it would be seen as part of the attraction (see Figure 12.6).

In Figure 12.6, an attempt has been made to reconstruct the relationships of the five single hearing impaired people in the study. Their missing hearing partners left the relationship either through death or divorce. The psychosocial constructions of this group were found to be 'a complaint', 'a sign of old age', 'an isolating problem', 'an unshared burden' and an 'intolerable burden'. Three out of the five couple perceptions in this group are at the negative end of the SSP spectrum.

In viewing all 16 psychosocial perceptions, it emerges that two negative perceptions on the SSP scale occurred when the hearing loss was mutually recognized before partnership acknowledgement. This is in comparison with five negative perceptions which emerged when the hearing loss occurred after partnership acknowledgement.

This may suggest that couples who mutually recognize 'deafness as a difference' within their partnership at the time of acknowledgement are more likely to acquire the 'quality factor' than relationships where the deafness is not part of the original attraction.

It is also of interest that seven out of the 16 couples perceived the deafness within their relationship as being an indifferent factor or at the positive end of the SSP scale. While this might indicate that there is a strong 'quality factor' operating, the actual findings are more complex. For example, it is shown that the second group of IF couples (7, 8, 9) are indifferent as a partial defence mechanism. In other words, an unconscious collusion takes place within these couples where the difficulties of being hearing impaired are not integrated within the marriage and had to be largely managed outside. There also seems to be a connection between the use of this 'splitting' defence and late marriages and/or late onset suggesting that the adaptability required is less likely to be present in later life.

Another trend in the analysis is that couples are likely to shift up towards the positive end of the axis after they have a certain time to get used to living with 'deafness as a difference' within their relationships. Couples are likely to shift towards the negative end of their perceptions at the time of family transitions such as the birth of a baby, children leaving home, or retirement.

It is hoped that the use of the chart of Shared Spousal Perceptions (Figure 12.1) will encourage helping professionals who work with couples where 'deafness is a difference' to become more sensitive to the very complex issues involved. More specifically that they will help both partners grow in acceptance and compassion and build the 'quality factor' of acceptance and integration in to their marriage.

The concluding chapter contains a summary of the nine most important arguments found in this book with a consideration of its limitations and some suggestions for further work.

CHAPTER 13

Conclusions

Introduction

This book has examined the challenges in relationships where one partner has a hearing impairment and the other hears normally. These challenges were studied within the couple relationship, and also within the surrounding social networks of which they were a part.

The term 'Hearing Differently' draws attention to the fact that the 11 couples and five single people who took part in this study did not belong completely to either the hearing or Deaf worlds. It was necessary for all of them to negotiate, forge, shape for themselves unique psycho/socio journeys which were somewhere in between these two sociological worlds, and which most accurately reflected their true inner selves. At the same time, they needed to be aware that there was a certain commonality of their experiences with other hearing impaired and Deaf people although this did *not* necessarily mean instant friendship unless the hearing loss was one of a group of friendship enhancing factors.

This process of negotiating one's journey could not be hurried, and had to be very patiently worked at as factors which facilitated these fledgling deaf/hearing identities and those which inhibited them were identified. The couples in this study were fortunate in that most of their hearing spouses, but not all, met the task of being co-monitors in this process. When this is not the case, counselling can help transform their relationship.

While the findings from this study are based on a small sample, those interviewed represent a very large range of people medically and developmentally. The 55 people, 28 of whom were children, came from a wide range of backgrounds in terms of class, education, ethnicity and religion. Although technically the sample may not be described as representative, that alone does not automatically define it as unrepresentative. We can learn from 'the micro' as embodied in family life, and make suggestions and generalizations which may apply to 'the macro' or society as a whole.

Hearing loss and family life

Hearing loss is widespread in our society. It affects every aspect of life where communication is necessary. There are ramifications for every level of daily life whether it is talking to one's partner in bed with the light out at night or being involved in high-level 'think tank' discussions in the board room.

Hearing loss is a very important social problem because the majority of people in our society will experience it at some time in their lives. Today as many as 7.5 million adults in the UK have a hearing impairment whose average loss exceeds 25 decibels. At least three-quarters of this group are over the age of 60. With this in mind, it is important to examine the projected rate of growth for elderly members of the population. For the year 2001, it has been estimated that 45 per cent of the population will be over 65 and 12 per cent will be aged over 75. Although old age is the leading aetiological factor in hearing impairment, NIHL (noise induced hearing loss) has been dramatically increasing. By the year 2015, the National Acoustics Laboratory of Australia predicts that 78 per cent of men and 25 per cent of women will be hearing impaired as a result of noise exposure.

Indeed this same article in *The Lancet* in September 1994 went so far as to suggest that hearing impairment, like failing eyesight, will in time reach epidemic proportions. This indicates that it is becoming increasingly important to study the ways in which hearing impairment makes its impact on intimate relationships.

Unquestionably, how to study the impact of hearing loss on relationships has continually baffled researchers. Much of the research to date has obscured many of the complexities involved in living with a hearing loss. The researcher's personal experience of profound hearing loss has suggested the considerable degree of complexity involved, particularly in the context of carrying out the roles of wife and mother. Furthermore, experiences as a social worker and counsellor suggested that the complexities in question might be more fruitfully explored and understood by adopting the technique of intensive repetitive interviewing, and by the use of a double focus: acquired hearing loss and family life.

By juxtaposing these two topics and by using the serial interviewing technique, it is shown how the former pathological picture of hearing impaired people, so widespread in the literature, was more likely to be a reflection of methodologies rather than reality. The limitations and imperfections of many former studies in the field of acquired hearing loss have become clear. By incorporating insights into the multi-faceted ambiguous nature of hearing loss together with an understanding of the anthropological approach as exemplified in the work of Elizabeth Bott, this study has succeeded in exposing many of the hidden shades of grey in the problem, as well as revealing a much more positive side of hearing loss and family life which other studies have not uncovered. It is hoped that hearing loss may never again be seen as a black or white issue of 'hearing' or 'not hearing'. The multi-faceted and ambiguous nature of hearing loss must be acknowledged and more adequate provision made for hearing impaired people.

In all these respects, this study has broken new ground as it has given a fuller, more comprehensive, shape to our understanding of the impact of hearing impairment on family life. The study could also be used as a model by other researchers, especially in the use of 'the life-cycle' approach to examine cross sections of family life where there is parental hearing loss. Although a limited approach in certain respects, it nevertheless provides a good framework for future qualitative family research into hearing impairment. A second theoretical construct which impinged on the entire study was an understanding of the systems perspective. People in this study were always viewed in context. The hearing loss was seen to belong to the couple, the family and the social network. It was never seen as a problem belonging solely to the individual as prescribed by the pathological model.

When examining some of the major strands and psychosocial insights which emerge from the study as a whole, and how they lead to recommendations for hearing therapy, research, and social policy, we need to keep in mind that their relevance has expanded with the formal implementation of community care proposals. Families and households will increasingly become primary settings for the care of people with disabilities. An effort has been made here to assess the particular needs not only of the people with the disabilities, but also of the family sub-systems, for example 'the couple' on the one hand, and 'the children' on the other.

1. The couple relationship: intimacy and the quality factor

The point has been made throughout that while 'deafness as a difference' can exacerbate marital difficulties, it is rarely if ever the sole cause of marital breakdown. Conversely, evidence indicates that a hearing loss can facilitate relationship development. This is because the various strategies required for comfortable conversation with a hearing impaired person, for example ETTA, and 'looking', and 'repeating', actually encourage the development of all relationships. Evidence for this has been found by Noller, who has noted that husbands who look at their wives when in conversation with them are 'high adjustment' husbands in that they are more likely to want to understand rather than to control their wives.

Using Sternberg's definition of intimacy as the emotional closeness component of a relationship, a related point is made that 'deafness as a difference' does not obstruct true intimacy, provided that both partners have genuine feelings of affection and regard for each other, and that more often than not, they are able to respond to each other's needs. With this foundation, couples can explore the various types of intimacy suggested by Professor Olson: emotional, social, intellectual, sexual, spiritual, and aesthetic.

A third point about marriage which emerged from the study is what may be called 'the quality factor'. It was put most succinctly by Theo aged 84 when she said:

> I'm glad that [I] did have patience [with my marriage to Will], because it was worth it, and I think today some people don't wait to see if somebody's worth it.

Certainly, a kind of fortitude and an ability to accept and integrate what comes is part of the quality factor. Parker also acknowledged this point with reference to the couples in her research:

> The pre-existing quality of the marriage and indeed, the personalities of the individuals involved, may be crucial in understanding what happens to couples after the onset of disability. Most marriages seem to survive, but whether or not they do is also related to the extent to which the partners are able to negotiate adjustment in their changed lives.

Lastly, the relationship and the partner needs to be revalued. This involves seeing the partner in the best possible light and acknowledging that not anyone could have done what they have done, and that, therefore, they are significant and special.

Not all the couples in this study were able to go through this process, and four marriage breakdowns did occur. It is significant that all four marriages broke down in Stage IV in the life-cycle. This fact confirms the literature's assertion that family tensions are the highest at this stage in that a massive transition is taking place as the children gradually become more adult and the parents attempt to rediscover what it is like to be a true couple again. Because it is such a vulnerable time, the teaching of very specific listening and communication skills is recommended, if they have not been learnt earlier, as there is enormous scope for misunderstandings. The teaching of such skills could be incorporated into NHS provision or through RELATE education programmes.

From primarily adult difficulties, we move to a discussion of the impact of hearing impairment on children. The literature suggests that children generally are not sympathetic when their parents are hearing impaired. This study suggests that the situation is more var able.

2. Management of hearing impairment and children

A second major strand to emerge was the importance of the response of children to one parent's hearing impairment. This was analysed using the family life-cycle approach. The experiences of the 11 couples interviewed suggested that hearing loss was easiest to manage when in fact there were no children as there was understandably less conflict between the ETTA factor (Effort, Time, Thought, Attention) required for one partner and the needs of the children. Generally, ETTA appeared to be the easiest to manage during middle childhood, Stage III, at a time when there is the least disruption to the family system, and children are identifying strongly with their parents. ETTA becomes most difficult when children were either joining the family at birth or leaving it as young adults. For example, when children are born, there is a loss of 'the couple' as the system becomes a small family. Traditionally it is the husband and new father who is most likely to feel excluded. If he happens also to be deaf, his feelings of exclusion are likely to be exacerbated. As we have seen, family tensions tend also to be very high during Stage V, the Adolescent Stage.

It was observed that step grand parenting combined with hearing loss could cause extra difficulties. It is possible that the more recent bonding of step grandparents will make competition and insecurity a stronger feature of relationships between generations.

The question still remains, how did the families in this book deviate from so called 'normal families' and what impact did the hearing impairment of one parent have on the children's lives?

It emerged that the hearing impairment of one parent, especially if it came as an unexpected crisis, could cause worry and/or resentment in their children. These negative feelings could be modified and even transformed by sensitive management of the children and the disability. Children could also be helped by being given continuing reassurance. This study suggested boys, eldest children, and children without siblings were in the most need of such reassurance because they appeared less able to illicit it naturally.

The main adjustment required of the children when communicating with their hearing impaired parents was to face them when speaking and to be 'lip-readable'. This sometimes meant that children had to first locate their parents in the house. Frustration was especially experienced when they found their parents behind locked doors, such as when they were in a bathroom or study, and had an added obstacle to overcome. Arthur, an adult child of Deaf parents, was the only one in the study who mentioned having responsibilities on behalf of his parents specifically in communicating with impatient 'officials'. He made it clear that he had not found this role unduly troublesome. There were no examples in the study of small children taking on adult responsibilities prematurely, a situation which has worried service providers as children are sometimes at risk when both parents are substantially hearing impaired.

There was considerable variation found in parental disclosure about hearing loss. It appeared that if disclosure took place when the children were quite young (3–5 years of age), the parents tended to emphasize 'responsibility' in their child rearing practices. On the other hand, if disclosure occurred slightly later (6–12 years of age), the parents appeared to be emphasizing a carefree childhood. In looking more closely at parent/child rapport, some parents were sensitive to a 'readiness factor' for discussions to take place, while others seemed aware of the need to create an appropriately 'close atmosphere' for such confidences.

Where reassuring discussions were not encouraged, there were a number of examples in the study of latency-aged children who appeared to want to share their parent's hearing loss, perhaps hoping that this identification would 'make things better'. One child faked a pure tones audiometric test and was actually given a hearing aid to wear; and another child, whose mother was traumatically deafened, appeared to isolate himself in his room in an apparent psychological simulation of deafness.

Throughout, grandchildren were observed as being just as capable as children in learning about adjustments to hearing loss, namely in making themselves lip-readable. The positive attitude of grandparents to both their grandchildren and their hearing loss facilitated this process.

3. Communication strategies: lip-reading and disclosure

While researchers have examined the cognitive components of lip-reading, the psychosocial components have long been neglected. Five psychosocial stress factors emerged: stress caused in encountering strangers, stress with unlipreadable children, stress for men generally who felt threatened or provoked by the intimacy required in the act of 'looking' in order to lip-read, stress in being forced to change long established marital communication patterns, and stress due to the forced 'looking' required when marital intimacy was experienced as frightening because of past failed relationships.

Findings also suggest that taking responsibility for lip-reading is an exercise in patience and courage on the part of both the hearing and the hearing impaired partner. Although feelings of irritation, frustration, and fatigue may be experienced on occasion, the more positive feelings of affection, respect and connectedness tend to prevail if a positive unconscious emotional 'fit' existed before the hearing loss was acquired.

The communication strategy of 'disclosure' was frequently used by study participants. It was used in a very discriminating manner rather than as a simplistic general policy of appropriate behaviour recommended by some professional rehabilitators. Some of the social factors which appeared to influence disclosure patterns were race, nationality, gender, religion, class and cultural values. Psychological and emotional factors which influenced decision making about disclosure were parental training, role expectations, personality of the speaker and the listener, immediacy of diagnosis, and concern for others. Lastly, environmental factors were mentioned such as when and where the question of 'disclosure' arose.

Thus it emerged that disclosure decisions made by the people in this study were based upon the interaction of numerous social, psychological, emotional, and environmental factors. This meant that they were most comfortable with a selective, thoughtful, sometimes intuitive disclosure policy, in effect very similar to hearing people generally in the management of the private details of their lives.

4. Evolving conceptions of care and ETTA

A fourth major strand concerned the specific nature of the 'care' provided for hearing impaired people by their partners, kin and friends. While it has been consistently maintained throughout this study that 'the help' which a hearing impaired partner receives from his hearing partner does not belong with traditional forms of caring, there are, nevertheless, connections with it, specifically in terms of the 'measurement' and 'cost' of care. For example, we have seen that the hearing partner may take on from time to time the roles of buffer, interpreter, mediator, prompter, advocate, monitor, and editor. These roles involved close proximity to hearing impaired people as found in 'tending' and 'psychological care'. However, unlike traditional 'tending' tasks, when the whole relationships of the couples in this study was viewed, the 'caring' that took place was reciprocal and mutual. In other words, relationships were interdependent because the care went both ways as illustrated in Figures 12.4 and 12.5. In this respect also this study departs from many earlier studies where the person being cared for has not been 'heard', although Barry and others are attempting to fill this gap.

The concept of ETTA (Effort, Time, Thought, Attention) has been introduced to signify 'the cost' in energy of care given as well as received. Hearing impaired people need 'access' to general conversation. While some people and cultures are naturally expressive and have a 'high involvement' manner with others, people from more restrained courteous cultures must think carefully about the extra energy expended so that a 'verbal ramp' is offered to a hearing impaired person. Problems may arise in the latter cultures where a certain type of intimate, emotional and personal communication is simply not part of cultural norms, unless people happen to be helping professionals and have integrated their professional values into their personal life.

There were some unexpected gender shifts in this study. More men appeared to be involved in 'caring', not in a traditional 'tending' sense, but in helping the hearing impaired person to ward off isolation in one way or another. Nearly all were quite happy to take on the communication roles described, while some maintained more secondary roles as 'watch dog'.

The other interesting shift was found in the stories of Max and Theo in that it was the widower, Max, who was surrounded by his 'caring' family, while it was the widow, Theo, who had almost more autonomy than she could manage.

5. Questioning some assumptions and labels

(a) As in every discipline, the literature in the deaf field holds to be true certain assumptions and labels until they are proven to be otherwise. The charts in Chapter 12 were developed in the hope that they would stimulate further thought about some of the medical/audiological and social policy assumptions which prevail. These show that the people in this study experienced no correlation between the time of onset and the degree of deafness with overall adjustment, and that 'care' was a reciprocal affair between the hearing impaired partner and the hearing partner.

(b) The findings here will call into question certain assumptions about prelingually deaf people, specifically the case of Arthur. Although theoretically his needs should have been different from the other people in the study with acquired hearing loss, his excellent command of spoken English as well as his use of BSL meant that his communication potential was equal to if not better than other hearing impaired people in the study. This suggests that 'labels' in the deaf field must be used with discrimination to ensure that they do justice to the complexities of the lives of individual deaf people.

(c) Up until this time most of the research in the deaf area has focused on how the experience of acquired deafness impoverishes the environment of hearing impaired people in comparison with people who hear. This book seeks to show that although some disadvantage does occur, nearly all of it can be compensated for by the acquisition of a psychologically healthy state of being for a hearing impaired person, by an informed and compassionate spouse, and by an informed and appropriately caring social network. This therefore suggests that the challenge for hearing people is to keep in mind that those with hearing loss are the same and different from themselves.

(d) Lastly, there are considerable discussions in the literature regarding the medical/individual model versus the social model of disability. This study draws from each model when appropriate and thrusts towards a fuller more comprehensive account of realities.

6. Rehabilitation worth

Another developing strand in the book was that hearing impaired people in the UK have not been given sufficient and/or appropriate guidance at the time they are diagnosed to help them cope with the multi-faceted ambiguous nature of acquired hearing loss which penetrates into the heart of all their intimate and social relationships. There appear to be three reasons for this connected with the individual, his social network, and societal norms generally.

First, people who acquire a hearing impairment carry within them the negative attitudes their socialization has taught them about deafness. Regardless of age, people still experience losing their hearing as an unexpected crisis, and it precipitates strong negative feelings, and sense of being noticed as different and stigmatized. As we have seen, these negative feelings lower self-esteem and confidence. This suggests that hearing impaired people themselves find it immensely difficult to make their needs known even if they are aware enough to understand their complexity and ambiguity and see themselves as credible friends. In this respect, hearing loss is an individual problem.

Secondly, this study indicates that kin, friends, and professionals who compose the social support network of the person with acquired hearing loss, are in fact in a very powerful position. This is because these people psychosocially construct the hearing impaired person's 'rehabilitation worth'.

Unfortunately, as we have seen, network members may often collude with the negativity already experienced by the person with acquired hearing loss rather than fight against this attitude, and a vicious circle is created resulting in the 'deafness as acquired oppression' described by Woolley (1994), Kyle (1993) and McKnight (1981). Informal or formal care managers often do not recognize the needs of people with acquired hearing loss because they are not expressed. There is often a defective assessment of needs even when they are assessed since most care managers are only aware of one or two aspects of the problem. When services are delivered through defective assessment, the same ignorance of the problem bedevils the relationship again, but on a lower level in the health care hierarchy. An example of this was Frank, whose wish to be informed about his hearing loss was thwarted by the technicians who fitted his hearing aid, because giving out such information at that level was against NHS policy.

Carers are also likely to discover that unless they understand the specific special needs of people with hearing loss and the greater possibility of communication breakdown, they are unlikely to obtain the full cooperation of people with hearing loss in their more general care.

Lastly, rather than being helpful, there are certain norms found in some cultures which work directly against the needs of hearing impaired people. A more general traditional norm in this instance is that people should live with their problems as best they can rather than seek help for understanding the multi-faceted nature of acquired hearing loss.

7. Social networks and hearing impairment

Although hearing impairment is often connected in the literature and in the imagination with isolation, it emerged that the majority of the study participants were not isolated. This was because most of them had learned, with the help of their partners, how to overcome the communication barriers and develop friendships in various ways. These will now be discussed.

(a) A number of people in the study, both hearing and hearing impaired partners, took a proactive approach in establishing their social network. From the beginning they sought to take charge of 'stigma management' in various ways. As we have seen, although Joy was unaware of any particular strategy, she did in fact follow one which included the following tactics: (1) she returned to live in the town where she grew up; this helped her to re-establish herself with old friends and formed the base of her network; (2) she quickly affirmed that she was the same person despite her deafness and had not lost her social skills; (3) she found that people could learn quickly how to speak to her by watching how her husband, Mike, operated; (4) doing things socially in couples and groups meant that ETTA and interpreting roles could be shared so that Mike could have a break if he wanted one; (5) they belonged to a self-help group.

(b) In examining the couples, it emerged strongly that those who were the best adjusted, all belonged to self-help groups of varying natures. Those represented were Crawley Hard of Hearing Group, the Break Through Trust, the Royal National Institute for the Deaf, LINK, Nigerian doctors in Britain, and the National Association of Deafened People (NADP). Each group had a different focus and provided different types of support, but there was the common similarity in that people with hearing impairments were accepted. Such groups were especially helpful for recently deafened people, or people who had experienced some other major transition such as a move or migration.

(c) For some people, their own family could make a most appropriate support or self-help group. The findings suggested that most families tried to provide support for their hearing impaired relations, but that they were continually bedevilled in this task because of the ambiguities involved. The best illustration of this was the widowed grandfather, Max. Although he longed to take part in conversation at the dinner table with his daughter's family, this was often difficult to do because of the conversational style which they adopted. Specifically, in Max's family, feelings of 'belonging' were generated by unstated meanings and being privy to the mundane details of everyday domestic life. When a hearing loss prevented their absorption by Max, the situation became more complex because of traditional English dislike of repeating so called 'trivia'.

Although such norms and habits are extremely difficult to change, awareness training programmes, for example in the need for ETTA, could be channelled through local RELATE organizations so that families might better understand the multi-faceted and ambiguous nature of hearing loss. There is also need for a revisioning of the two major communicating strategies required, 'repeating' and 'looking', so that they may be seen as an enhancement to conversation rather than an obligation and a threat to established norms (Paxman, 1998).

(d) All the people in the book had contact with professionals who were also part of their social networks. Teachers and social workers were seen to be the least helpful as they were connected with past oppression and disapproval of BSL. Doctors were seen as helpful especially if they understood their value to their hearing impaired patients despite the fact that they could not cure them. Clergymen were generally seen as helpful facilitators.

Very few of the study participants had actually met a Hearing Therapist, which is not surprising considering the small numbers that have been trained. A way forward here will be discussed in the next section.

8. Recommendations for social policy

It is obvious that there is no one solution for helping people with acquired hearing loss become more integrated within their families and within society. However, some recommendations may be made. First, a multi-disciplinary holistic approach must be adopted when working with hearing impaired people because of the multifaceted nature of the problem. This may be done partly by upgrading the training of Hearing Therapists so that they receive a more rigorous foundation in the theoretical aspects of their profession away from the medical model towards a deeper understanding of the systems perspective and psychosocial aspects of hearing loss.

Other professionals working with people with acquired hearing loss must put rivalry aside and insist on greater cooperation across the services of education, the national health service and social services. Ideally an institute should be established where a multi-disciplinary holistic approach could be employed and counselling, training, and research into acquired hearing loss take place. Such developments would be in line with the original recommendations made to the DHSS by their subcommittee, ACSHIP, which were unfortunately so neglected when hearing therapy was established in 1978. Much also may be learned from the experiences of Sweden, Germany, Denmark, and the USA.

Such developments need not wait for the actions of politicians. Hearing impaired people themselves have a crucial role to play in helping to change ideas, services, and policies in ways which suit them.

In other words due to the importance of developing a group iden-tity to facilitate the creation of a platform at local and national levels, it would be of enormous benefit if self-help groups could be estab-lished, run by executive committees composed of hearing impaired people with the support of hearing people. This would help hearing impaired people in a number of areas. First, they would find support and understanding by interacting with other hearing impaired people. Secondly, their sense of' 'rehabilitation worth' would rise as they became more accepting and knowledgeable about hearing impairment. Thirdly, with acceptance and knowledge comes respon-sibility, and hopefully the capacity to communicate to others the complex nature of hearing loss. Fourthly, awareness and training programmes need to be introduced so that families may learn how to transform aspects of their attitudes and domestic culture which cause their hearing impaired members particular frustration. Rocky Stone, the founder of SHHH (Self Help for Hearing Impaired People) in the USA had this to say about the benefits of a self-help approach:

> Most of us recognize that human understanding is possible only as long as chan-nels of communication are kept open. Unless we can communicate with our neighbour we have little chance of understanding him, or vice versa. When there is a breakdown in the communications process, such as loss of hearing in one of the participants, not only good will but knowledge becomes important. We have to find new ways to communicate. We have to do this while retaining confidence that the human spirit is stronger than anything that can happen to it. We have only lost our hearing ... not our humanness.
>
> Once we get this into perspective, we can generate the courage to go on. And we go on with others. We are engaged in 'Self Help'. We are pulling together ... all crew, no passengers. And though the race be difficult, we feel better already.
>
> Thousands of hard of hearing people throughout the USA, in Canada and Australia, have made a decision about themselves. They are learning, growing, asserting ... they are Self Help in Action.

9. Recommendations for further research

With regard to future research, there is much to be done. On a general level, more research needs to focus on families and how they respond to a family member who has a sensory loss such as hearing impairment as there are so many ambiguities involved, and because communication is so central an issue in family life. This could be done by building on the framework established in this study using the family life-cycle although the family life course could also be used.

Most of the couples in this study were middle-class and well educated. A study along similar lines, but where there is more disad-vantage, is recommended. We need to know more about what happens in families who experience financial deprivation or who face other difficulties in responding to this challenge.

More substantial research on lip-reading is needed to tease out the impact of various social factors such as culture, gender, ethnicity, personality, personal history, and feelings about the person speaking.

Another area which this study suggests is that of more research into the lives of elderly people and their friendships, as nearly 50 per cent are hearing impaired and many appear to suffer because of this.

The paradox seems to be that when one discovers answers for understanding distinctive relationships, the same knowledge may be applied for all couple/family relationships in that it is impossible to live together with out confronting 'differences' whether it is gender, personality, nationality or hearing loss.

Appendices

Appendix A: Who were the people?

The nucleus group of couples for this study was discovered at the 1988 AGM of the National Association of Deafened People. Other people were found through sponsors known to me through the membership of certain organizations: The Committee for Staff and Students with Disabilities at the Institute of Education University of London, the Women's Workshop on Qualitative Family and Household Research, and the Church of England. This situation very much confirmed Bott's experience that personal sponsorship lead to committed respondents.

While some experts in the deaf field would argue that a study sample should consist of either prelingually deaf people or people with acquired hearing loss, I was interested in observing a group of people that represented a continuum. In other words, the range rather than the degree of deafness was the important factor.

Although the 11 couples and five single people in the study had hearing impairment as a common factor, there was considerable variety in other social factors. This was seen to be appropriate in order to avoid the stereotypical view that hearing impaired people are a homogeneous group.

For example, of the 27 adults in the study, 11 could be considered members of social class I on the Registrar General's classification; nine of social class II, six of social class III, none of social class IV, and one of social class V. Also related to class was the fact that all but one of the 11 couples were dual career couples in the sense that both husband and wife had regular earnings.

Not surprisingly, class seemed closely connected with years of education. Eleven people had received a professional qualification and/or an advanced graduate education; six had received BAs and six had done some A levels and/or an additional diploma. Four people had received a secondary education or less. The small number who did not have general educational qualifications on a high level was in practice very articulate.

Ethnicity, religion and gender were also social factors examined. The nationalities represented included English, Scottish, French, Nigerian and American. The religious affiliations represented were Anglicans, Methodists, Presbyterians and Jews. With respect to gender, of the 16 hearing impaired people who took part in the study, eight were men and eight were women, though half the women belonged to the single hearing impaired group, among whom there was only one man.

There was also considerable variety among the couples with regard to degree of hearing impairment. Of the 16 hearing impaired people in the study, six were diagnosed by their audiologists using a pure tones test as having profound to total hearing losses; four people were diagnosed as being severely hearing impaired; three people had moderate to severe hearing losses; and three people were diagnosed as having mild to moderate losses. There were people in the study who were born deaf and/or acquired a form of deafness later in life. Different types of deafness were represented. Most of the sample had sensorineural losses, but one had a conductive loss, specifically otosclerosis. The rapidity of loss varied: three hearing impaired subjects had experienced sudden traumatic loss, while the remaining 13 experienced their losses gradually.

In selecting couples, formal marriage was not considered an essential criterion, though in the event all but two were married. A factor which was of more concern was the 'stability' perceived in the relationship. Did the couple possess the equilibrium needed to withstand sustained involvement with an outside researcher along with a genuine interest in exploring the topics under discussion; or was there a certain fragility present that made the possibility of early withdrawal likely, for example a suspicious, hostile or prickly couple presentation?

Interviewing the people

These concerns made it imperative from the outset to communicate the demanding nature of repeated intensive interviewing. An important aspect of establishing the trust required to sustain people's involvement in the interviewing process was an open discussion of the interviewer's own family history and hearing impairment.

Understandably, the open-ended nature of the initial questioning resulted in some anxiety. Therefore, guidelines for discussion were drawn up and presented to each couple at the initial interview. They were helpful to most, although one couple refused to see them for fear they would inhibit rather than help the sharing process.

Also included in the interviewing process were marital exercises devised by the researcher from a guide for marriage enrichment (Garland, 1983). While the original purpose of the exercises was to help couples improve their ability to communicate openly, solve problems and manage conflict, their use in this study was to stimulate discussion in more intimate areas of married life. These were based on a 'developmental' framework (Duvall and Hill, 1948).

Initially the decision was made to interview both husband and wife exploring deeper issues of conflict and differences, using listening techniques I learnt in RELATE counselling training, and also known to social researchers. They provided an atmosphere in which different issues could be safely explored. Also structured into the sessions from the beginning were expectations that couples would be interviewed together and separately.

All the interviews took place in the people's homes. The exact positioning of the interviews was important since effective communication was best when sitting relatively close together in full view of each other's faces. Experience suggested that the most suitable place was the kitchen or dining room table.

The interviews were made as egalitarian as possible to avoid distortion and 'interviewer bias'. One method to help this process was found by devising an Agreement Form. The people in the study were shown the form and asked to sign it if they wished. The form discussed confidentiality, procedures about publication of findings, expectations of individual interviews, and premature withdrawal from the study. Most of the couples signed it at the second session when they began to understand what was being expected of them. Others preferred to wait until the interviewing was finished before signing. One couple, both members of the legal profession, rewrote parts of it and their suggestions were incorporated. Some couples expressed the concern that the Agreement Form was making everything too formal. Others understood the practical and ethical value of it in case some aspect of the study was misunderstood or misheard. The provision of a file for the papers required helped to ensure that the exercise was taken seriously by everyone involved.

The continuing interviews

The correct pacing of interviews with each couple was important to establish. Because there was so much variation, it took a little time to find the most appropriate speed which included both hearing and hearing impaired partners and the hearing impaired researcher.

Couples were also asked how they felt about the gender and the disability balance in the interview. For example men were asked how they felt talking with two women and the hearing partners were asked how they felt talking to two hearing impaired people.

The length of the interview was another point negotiated. As the researcher travelled by public transport, some interviews ended abruptly since there was a train to catch. Some couples complained that one hour was not long enough since they were 'just warming up'. When this happened, the session could sometimes be rearranged to one and a half hours. With the vulnerability and diversity present, it seemed essential not to go over the time limit, and also to honour the psychological defences in use.

The number of interviews was not directly contested. Once the interviews were established, there seemed a gradual shift from 'public accounts' to 'private accounts'. Only the first couple withdrew prematurely. The reason given was that the hearing impaired wife had taken on responsibilities which she perceived as being incompatible with her role as respondent in the study.

Couples appeared to participate in the study for different reasons. A number of couples approached it as a way to evaluate themselves as Bott (1957) also found. They were aware of a certain level of risk and managed to keep the balance between over and under risking in what they revealed. Others were a little more anxious and expressed concern that some of the questions asked might spoil something 'special' which they had as a family or a couple.

Research tools

In this study tape recordings and the resulting typed transcripts were vital. Apart from providing a full record of the interviews and a source from which illustrative material could be drawn, as time went on they also aided recall and that which had not been heard or was considered inconsequential at the first reading. This helped to develop a more sensitive and accurate interviewing technique.

Five secretaries worked on the transcripts. The work of the secretaries was partly paid for from a grant received from the LSE graduate school. Hand notes of every session were also taken and typed up afterwards. They acted as an immediate reminder of what had taken place. They also showed more quickly what had been covered and in what direction the interviews were going.

Initially it was hoped that a number of interviews would be videoed. However, it soon became apparent that the size of the equipment and the distances involved made this plan impractical. Fortunately, it was possible to video one couple twice and this has since been used for demonstration purposes.

British Sign Language was not learned, since as it emerged it was not relevant for this specific study as only once couple used it on a regular basis. They were surprised at my lack of skill in BSL and would probably have withdrawn at that point except for the fact that their sponsor had given the researcher an excellent recommendation.

Appendix B: Profiles of the study's 11 couples and five individuals

Joy (HI) and Mike (H)

Joy (60) and Mike (60) have been married 30 years. Mike works for a printing firm. Before Joy was deafened, they ran a business together. Joy was deafened at 37 years of age from meningitis. Although in business with her husband at the time she was deafened, she later obtained a job as a dinner lady in a school cafeteria. They have one son James, now 30, who has recently married. Joy was an early cochlear implantee. She lip-reads and is presently enrolled in a

British Sign Language course. This couple represented Stage VI in the Middle Years in the family life-cycle.

Julia (H) and Sam (HI)

Sam (41) was deafened from drug toxicity at 18 years of age. He was, nevertheless, able to complete a science degree at the university where he met Julia (33). Sam is a computer programmer for a City company and Julia co-directs a textile business. They have no children and have been living together for ten years. Sam wears no hearing aid and relies on lip-reading and his partner's interpretation. He knows BSL and some finger spelling, having taught briefly at a School for the Deaf. This couple represented partners without children in Stage I in the family life-cycle.

Barbara (HI) and Ben (H)

Barbara (40) was severely hearing impaired at birth resulting from her mother's rubella. She met Ben (39) after both had qualified as professional people in the same field. They have been married for ten years and have two children, Louise (10) and Jonathan (9) who were interviewed. Barbara has since become an administrator in a national charity. She is an excellent lip-reader and wears both behind the ear aid as well as a box aid on occasion. This family represented Stage III in the family life-cycle.

Sarah (H) and Joe (HI)

Sarah (47) and Joe have been married for seven years. Both have children and grandchildren from former marriages. Sarah has a daughter and two grandsons. Joe has two sons who were estranged, but have recently become reunited with him. Joe lost much of his hearing as a baby from diphtheria. Today he has severe loss, wears two hearing aids and is an excellent lipreader. He has his own design business. Sarah is employed as a lipreading teacher by her local authority. They represent Stage VI or the Middle Years of the Family Life Cycle.

Kay (H) and Henry (HI)

Kay (41) and Henry (39) have been married for just over six years. Henry was born with a severe hearing loss resulting from his mother's rubella. He wears two hearing aids and is an excellent lip-reader. This couple represented Stage II in the family life-cycle as they have two children, Clive (4) and Christy (1). At the time of the interviews, Kay, an experienced teacher, and Henry were finishing up their training for the ordained ministry in the church of England and were looking forward to leaving college and serving in their first parish church. Henry had recently completed Stage I in BSL.

Gwen (H) and Arthur (HI)

Gwen (27) and Arthur (26) were in Stage I and the only newly weds in the study as they had been married for just over one year when the interviews began. Arthur has a profound hearing loss and grew up as a member of a Deaf family. He wears two hearing aids, lip-reads and Signs with fluency. Gwen worked as a primary school teacher and gave birth to a son during the interview period. Consequently, Arthur has decided to give up his studies and take up a civil service position.

Anne (HI) and Adam (H)

Anne (38) and Adam (42) have been married for 18 years. They represented Stage III and IV in the family life-cycle as their children Jane and Rupert were 11 and 13 years of age respectively. Anne had very recently been diagnosed as having mild/moderate sensorin-ueral bilateral hearing loss. She did not wear an aid nor did she lip-read. She has been working as a social researcher for some time while Adam was the head of the business department in a college of further education. Jane and Rupert were also interviewed.

Simone (H) and Frank (HI)

Simone (63) and Frank (64) had been married for 39 years and repre-sented Stage VI in the family life-cycle. Eight years earlier, Frank was diagnosed as having a mild/moderate sensorinural bilateral hearing loss. He varied in wearing one, sometimes two hearing aids, but does not lip-read. Simone, who is French, had recently retired as the head of the French department of a secondary school. At the time of the interviews, Frank was nearing retirement as a Professor of History and Administrator in a London University. They had two adult chil-dren, five grandchildren, as well as Simone's elderly parents to look after during the holiday periods in France.

Anthony (HI) and Clare (H)

Anthony (37) and Clare (30) have been married for ten years and have three school aged children. They were in Stage III of the family life-cycle. Anthony and Clare are African. They came to the UK for Anthony to be rehabilitated after he was deafened from drugs given to save his life when complications arose during an appendicectomy operation. Anthony, a doctor, was eventually able to retrain as a pathologist while Clare worked as an accommodations' officer for their local council. Anthony and Clare are the one couple in the study who attended the Link Centre, the British Centre for Deafened People in Eastbourne. Anthony wears a hearing aid with a masker because of his tinnitus. Anthony and Clare's eldest son was also interviewed.

Mary (H) and Robert (HI)

Mary (68) and Robert (71) were retired teachers with four adult children and six grandchildren. They represented Stage VII in the family life-cycle. Robert had contracted Menière's Disease just before he retired. At the same time, the family experienced two other crises: Mary and Robert had a Down's Syndrome grandchild and their youngest son had a mental breakdown. Robert coped by becoming proficient in the use of a radio microphone although he continued to suffer from vertigo. Mary trained late in life as a 'special needs' teacher. She has taken early retirement so as to be more available to her family. Three of their four children were also interviewed.

Rachel (H) and Richard (H)

Rachel (46) and Richard (50) had been married for 23 years. They have two sons, John and William, who were in the process of leaving home. Consequently, this family represented Stage V in the family life-cycle. Rachel had contracted otosclerosis when she was 26, a condition inherited from her father. She wears two hearing aids, and has been operated on for her condition. She does not lip-read. Richard runs a consultancy agency and Rachel is a sociology lecturer.

Grace (HI)

Sue (70) is single and divorced, having previously been married to her husband for 22 years. She maintained a business partnership with him which involved her as the decorator in conversions of old flats. She had gradually acquired her profound hearing loss which had been inherited from her mother. She is active in deaf advocacy work, but has no children.

Christine (HI)

Christine (70) is also single and divorced. Her former husband, a doctor, left her for another woman, and eventually died. Christine now has three sons and 8 grandchildren who she sees regularly. Christine was gradually deafened, a condition thought to be caused by pneumonia in childhood. She has a cochlear implant, lip-reads and uses sign language (ASL). At 50 she retrained as a rehabilitation counsellor and researcher. She has retired from counselling, but continues to do research.

Martha (HI)

Martha (55) is a single mother and has two adult children. She blames her severe hearing loss on scarlet fever which she had as a child. She lives with her son, a niece, and a dog. The father of her children left her many years ago and she is presently on social security. She wears one hearing aid with difficulty. She suffers from periods of depression.

Theo (HI)

Theo (84) has been a widow for the last three years. Before her retirement at 71, she was the headmistress of a private primary school. She has one son and three grandchildren. She has a mild/moderate hearing loss and wears one hearing aid. She has never been to a hospital to be properly tested.

Max (HI)

Max (81) has been a widower for the last seven years. He has two adult daughters and seven grandchildren. He was formerly the headmaster of a large comprehensive secondary school in London and was once the chairperson of his Union. He has a mild/moderate hearing loss, presbycusis, and wears one hearing aid. His two daughters, son in law and one grandson were also interviewed.

All the people in the study lived in London with the exception of Gwen and Arthur who lived in a provincial city in the South of England.

Appendix C

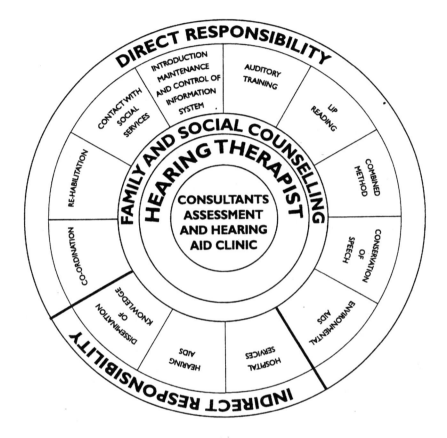

Figure A1. The direct and indirect responsibilities of the Hearing Therapist as stipulated in the 1975 ACSHIP Report.

Notes

1. The term 'hearing impairment' has been used to include all people with any degree of hearing loss from slight to profound. Despite the term's unpopularity in certain quarters, hearing impairment is used descriptively in this book because (1) no more appropriate term has presented itself and (2) it represents the comprehensive range of the people's hearing loss who took part in this study. These people must be seen as being neither totally deaf nor totally hearing, if not in the physical sense, certainly in the psychological one.

2. The use of the higher case 'D' will be used for the rest of this book following in the Woodward (1972) tradition.

3. The ETTA (Effort, Time, Thought and Attention) concept includes all strategies in the literature for helping hearing impaired people to lip-read. For example, it includes the importance of knowing that (a) for the speaker to be standing in front of a window makes lip-reading difficult; (b) being in a noisy environment makes using hearing aids difficult; (c) hands covering any part of the face makes lip-reading difficult; (d) rooms where there are many soft furnishings facilitate hearing and listening as they will absorb any 'echo' that is in the room.

4. This principle of networking has been conceptualized in DMEN (Developing Mutually Enhancing Networks) because of its importance. Couples who have many differences may, if they are not careful, develop two completely different social networks which have the effect of working against the couple's cohesion rather than for it. DMEN suggests that a strategic effort may need to be made to ensure that a certain number of friends are mutually shared and valued.

5. Looking at the role of professionals in the lives of hearing impaired people will be completed in Chapter 11 where there will be a discussion of the role of Hearing Therapists and professionals who are not formal rehabilitators. The importance of social networks in the lives of the study participants may also be seen in Chapter 12.

6. Olson and his colleagues discovered that appropriate amounts of the three family dimensions – adaptability, cohesion and a facili-

tating communication – were crucial in developing optimally functioning families. By adaptability is meant the ability of marital/family systems to change their power structure, role relationships and relationship rules in response to situational and developmental stress. Cohesion is about how close family members feel emotionally to one another. The facilitating communication helps to alter these factors when needed.

7. The term 'family/household therapeutic alliance' is not reintroducing the medical or therapeutic model, but in fact is maintaining professional terminology already used, for example the use of the term 'hearing therapy'. The term also draws attention once again to the fact that hearing loss belongs to everyone in a family and a household and not just to the individual.

8. D.S.R. Garland's book, *Working with Couples for Marriage Enrichment*, is one of many which help couples assess and improve their marriages while taking part in group and couple sessions.

* H = Hearing and HI = Hearing impaired.

Bibliography

Abrams P (1980) Social change, social networks and neighbourhood care. Social Work Services 22:12–23, February.

Ackehurst S (1989) Broken Silence. Sydney: William Collins Ltd.

Adams RG (1986) Secondary friendship networks and psychological well-being among elderly women. Activities, Adaptation and Aging 8: 59–72.

Ageing (1990) A Report from the Board for Social Responsibility. London: Church House Publishing.

Ainlay S, Becker G, Coleman LM (eds) (1986) The Dilemma of Difference: A Multidisciplinary View of Stigma. London: Plenum Press.

Ainsworth MDA (1982) Attachment: retrospect and prospect. In CM Parkes, J Stevenson-Hinde (eds), The Place of Attachment in Human Behaviours. New York: Basic Books, 3–30.

Allan G (1979) A Sociology of Friendship and Kinship. London: Allen & Unwin.

Allan G (1989) Friendships: Developing a Sociological Perspective. London: Harvester Wheatsheaf.

Alpiner JG (1980) Aural Rehabilitation for Adults. In RL Schow, MA Nerbonne (eds), Introduction to Aural Rehabilitation. Baltimore: University Park Press.

Appleton PL, Minchom PE (1991) Models of parent partnership and child development centres: Scottish Concern, Journal of Children's Bureau, Scottish Group. Special Issue, Parents with Disabilities: 54–68.

Argyle M, Lalljee M, Cook M (1968) The effects of visibility on interaction in a dyad. Human Relations 21: 3–18.

Arling D (1976) Resistance to isolation among elderly widows. International Journal for Ageing and Human Development 7: 67–86.

Ashley P (1985) Deafness in the family. In H Orlans (ed.), Adjustment to Adult Hearing Loss. London: Taylor & Francis, 71–82.

Askham J (1984) Identity and Stability in Marriage. Cambridge: Cambridge University Press.

Attwell N, Watts F (1987) Hearing therapy and hearing loss. In J Kyle (ed.), Adjustment to Acquired Hearing Loss. Bristol: Centre for Deaf Studies, 231–7.

Baldwin S (1985) The Cost of Caring: Families with Disabled Children. London: Routledge & Kegan Paul.

Balint M (1996) The Doctor, His Patient, and the Illness. New York: International Universities Press Inc.

Ballantyne J (1975) Advisory Committee on Services for Hearing Impaired People, Rehabilitation of the Adult Deaf, A Survey, September.

Barbara A (1989) Marriage Across Frontiers. Philadelphia: Mullet Lingual Matters Ltd.

Barratte S, Burke C, Dived K, Stedman M, Ravel H (1999) Theoretical bases in relation to race, ethnicity and culture in family therapy training. Kent: The Invitee Press, 4–12.

Barry J (1995) Care-needs and care-receivers: view from the margins. In R Edwards, J Ribbons (Des) Women Studies International Form-Special Issue 18: 245–383.

Bart P (1970) Mother Portion's Complaint, Transaction 8: 69–74.

Beattie JA (1981) Social Aspects of Acquired Hearing Loss in Adults: a report on the research project funded by the Department of Health and Social Security and carried out in the Postgraduate School of Applied Social Studies, University of Bradford 1978–1981.

Beck R (1991) The hearing impaired psychotherapist: implications for process and practice. Clinical Social Work Journal 19(4): 417–26.

Becker G (1980) Growing Old in Silence. London: University of California Press.

Bengston VL, Cutler NE (1976) Generations and intergenerational relations. In RH Burstock, E Shines (Des) Handbook of Ageing and the Social Sciences. New York: Van Nostrand Reinhold.

Berger PL, Kellner H (1964) Marriage and the construction of reality, Diagnose, 1–23.

Bernard J (1982) The Future of Marriage. London: Yale University Press.

Blau P (1967) Exchange and Power in Social Life. New York: John Wiley and Sons.

Blaxter M (1976) The Meaning of Disability, A Sociological Study of Impairment. London: Heinemann.

Blumer H (1962) Symbolic Interactions: Perspective and Method. Englewood Cliffs N.J.: Prentice Hall.

Boone M (1993) Equalling Access to Sound. Reprinted from Your Church, for SHHH Publications, Bethesda, MD, February.

Boss P (1991) Ambiguous loss. In F Walsh, M McGoldrick (eds), Living Beyond Loss. London: W.W. Norton & Co., 164–75.

Bott E (1957) Family and Social Network. London: Tavistock Publications Ltd.

Bowen M (1991) Family reaction to death. In F Walsh, M McGoldrick (eds), Living Beyond Loss, Death in the Family. London: W.W. Norton & Co., 79–92.

Bowlby J (1969) Attachment and Loss, Vol. I. Harmondsworth: Penguin Books Ltd.

Bowlby J (1975) Attachment theory, separation anxiety and mourning. In DA Hamburg, HKM Brodie (eds), American Handbook of Psychiatry, New Psychiatric Frontier. New York: Basic Books 6: 292–309.

Brain R (1976) Friends and Lovers. London: Hart-Davis MacGibbon.

Brierley P (1991) Christian England: What the 1989 English Church Census Reveals. London: MARC Europe.

Broderick CB (1988) Healing members and relationships in the intimate network. In RM Milardo (ed.) Families and Social Networks. London: Sage Publications, 221–34.

Broderick CB (1993) Understanding Family Process, Basics of Family Systems Theory. London: Sage Publications.

Brown, D (1981) All in the Family. Disabled USA 4(3): 30–5.

British Society of Hearing Therapists (NDG) Hearing Therapy Career Leaflet, c/o MSF Regional Centre, Dane O'Coy's Road. Bishop's Stortford, Herts CM23 2JN.

Bulmer M. (1986) Neighbours: The Work of Philip Abrams. Cambridge: Cambridge University Press.

Bulmer M (1987) The Social Basis of Community Care. London: Unwin Hyman.

Burgoyne J (1985) Cohabitation and Contemporary Family Life. ESRC end-of-grant report.

Burgoyne J, Clark D (1984) Making a Go of It: A Study of Stepfamilies in Sheffield. London: Routledge & Kegan Paul.

Burgoyne J, Ormond R, Richards M (1987) Divorce Matters. Harmondsworth: Penguin.

Burns CL, Farina A (1984) Social competence and adjustment. Journal of Social and Personal Relationships 1: 99–113.

Byng-Hall S (1985) Resolving distance conflicts. In AS Gurman (ed.), Casebook of Marital Therapy. London: The Guilford Press, 1–19.

Campling J (ed.) (1981) Images of Ourselves. London: Routledge & Kegan Paul.

Chronically Sick and Disabled Person's Act (1970) Research and Development Work on Equipment for the Disabled (H.C.299)(102299730) 1–16.

Church J (ed.) (1995) Social Trends 25 Edition. London: HMSO Central Statistical Office 22, Table 1.13.

Clark D, Haldane D (1990) Wedlock: Intervention and Research in Marriage. Cambridge: Polity Press in Association with Basil Blackwell.

Clark M, Anderson BG (1980) Loneliness and old age. In J Hart, JR Andy, YA Cohen (Des), The Anatomy of Loneliness. New York: International University Press.

Clulow C (1995) Marriage: a new millennium? In C Clulow (ed.), Women, Men and Marriage. London: Sheldon Press, 145–59.

Clulow C, Mattinson J (1989) Marriage Inside Out. London: Penguin.

Clulow C, Vincent C (1987) In the Child's Best Interest. London: Tavistock Publications.

Cohen CI, Rajkowski H (1982) What's in a friend? substantive and theoretical issues, The Gerontologist 22: 261–6.

Cohen G (1987) Social Change and the Life Course. London: Tavistock Publications.

Cohen LH (1994) Train Go Sorry, Inside a Deaf World. New York: Houghton Mifflin Co.

Cohen MB (1974) Personal identity and sexual identity. In JB Miller (ed.), Psychoanalysis and Women, Harmondsworth: Penguin Books.

Commission on Rehabilitation Counsellor Certification (2000) CRC Certification Guide, Rolling Meadows, Illinois 60008.

Cooper D (1972) The Death of the Family. Harmondsworth: Penguin.

Corker M (1994) Counselling – The Deaf Challenge. London: Jessica Kingsley Publishers.

Cornwell J (1984) Hard-Earned Lives. London: Tavistock Publications.

Cornwell J, Gearing B (1989) Doing biographical reviews with older people, Oral History 17(1): 36–43.

Cowen CP et al. (1985) Transition to parenthood: his, hers and theirs. Journal of Family Issues 6(4): 451–81.

Cowrie R, Douglas-Cowrie E (1987) What happens when a member of a family acquires a hearing loss. Paper delivered to the British Society for the Advancement of Science, Belfast.

Criswell EC (1979) Deaf Action Centre's Senior Citizen Program, Journal of Rehabilitation of the Deaf 12: 36–40.

Cunningham-Burley S (1987) The experience of grandfatherhood. In C Lewis, M O'Brien (eds), Reassessing Fatherhood. London: Sage, 91–108.

DHSS-ACSHIP (1975) Department of Health and Social Security Advisory Committee on Services for Hearing Impaired People, Report of a Sub-committee Appointed to Consider the Rehabilitation of the Adult Hearing Impaired. London: HMSO.

DHSS-Circular HC(78)11) (1978) Department of Health and Social Security, Health Services Development: Appointment of Hearing Therapists. London: HMSO.

Dickens WJ, Perlman D (1981) Friendship over the lifecycle. In S Duck, R Gilmour (eds), Personal Relationships 2: Developing Personal Relationships. London: Academic Press.

Dicks HV (1967) Marital Tensions. London: Routledge & Kegan Paul.

Dominian J (1975) Cycles of Affirmation. London: Darton, Longman & Todd.

Dominian J (1985) Values in marriage: change and continuity. In W Dryden (ed.), Marital Therapy in Britain. London: Harper & Row 1: 34–50.

Dominian J, Mansfield P, Dormor D, McAllister F (1991) Marital Breakdown and the Health of the Nation, A Response to the Government's Consultative Document for Health in England: One Plus One Marriage and Partnership Research.

Dormor D (1990) Marriage and Partnership, One Plus One, Marriage and Partnership Research.

Doucet A (1995) Gender Differences and Gender Equality and Care: Towards Understanding Gendered Labour in British Dual Earner Households. Unpublished Doctoral Dissertation. Faculty of Social and Political Sciences, University of Cambridge.

Downing C (1990) Psyche's Sisters. New York: Continuum.

Doyle J, Paludi M (1991) Sex and Gender. Dubuque, Iowa: Wm C. Brown.

Doyle L, Gough I (1986) A Theory of Human Needs. London: Macmillan.

Dueck E, FRCS (1984) Interview at Guys Hospital, St Thomas Street. 10 May.

Duvall EM, Hill RL (1948) Report of the Committee on Dynamics of Family Interaction, National Conference on Family Life, Washington DC.

Earhart E, Sporakowski MJ (1984) Special Issue: The Family with Handicapped Members. Family Relations 33(1).

Eichler M (1981) Power, dependency, love and the sexual division of labour. Women's Studies International Quarterly 4(2): 201-19.

Elliott H (1978) Shifting Gears. Paper presented at a Workshop for Deafened Adults of the Hearing Society for the Bay Area and the Deaf Counselling Advocacy and Referral Agency.

Ellyson SL (1978) Visual Behaviour Exhibited by Males Differing as to Interpersonal Control Orientation in One- and Two-way Communication Systems. Unpublished master thesis, 1974. Cited in Harper RG, Wiens AN, Matarazzo JD, Nonverbal Communication: The State of the Art. New York: Wiley.

Emerson JP (1970) Nothing unusual is happening. In T Shibutani (ed.), Human Nature and Collective Behaviour. Englewood Cliffs, NJ.: Prentice Hall.

Erikson EH (1965) Childhood and Society. London: Paladin Grafton Books.

Etherington K (2000) Letter from the Course Coordinator of the Diploma/MSc in Counselling in Primary Care/Health Settings, University of Bristol Counselling

Programme, Graduate School of Education, 8–10 Berkeley Square, Clifton, Bristol BS8 1HH.

Evening Standard (1999) Deaf before her time, 20 July.

Finch J (1989) Family Obligations and Social Change. Cambridge: Polity Press.

Finch J, Groves D (1980) Community care and the family: a case for equal opportunities? Journal of Social Policy. Cambridge: Cambridge University Press.

Fischer CS (1982) To Dwell Among Friends: Personal Networks in Town and City. Chicago: University of Chicago Press.

Fishman S (1959) Amputee needs, frustrations, and behaviour. Rehabilitation Literature 20: 328.

Fitzpatrick MA (1988) Between Husbands and Wives. London: Sage Publications.

Fortes M (1969) Kinship and the Social Order. Chicago: Aldine.

Foster S (1989) Social alienation and peer identification: a study of the social construction of deafness. Human Organisation 48(3): 226–35.

Fraiberg SH (1959) The Magic Years. New York: Charles Scribner's Sons.

Frankel BG, Turner RJ (1983) Psychological Adjustment in Chronic Disability: Canadian Journal of Sociology 8: 273-291.

Freid M (1962) Grieving for a lost home. In LJ Duhl (ed.), The Environment of the Metropolis, Basic Books: New York.

French JRP Jr, Raven BH (1962) The bases of social power. In D Cartwright, A Zander (eds), Group Dynamics. Evanston Ill: Row Peterson 607–23.

Fromberg J (1989) Psychotherapeutic Cures at Bad Berleburg-Holistic Therapy for the Psychological Stability of Hearing-Impaired Persons. Rehabilitation Schwerhoriger, Ertaubter und Gehorloser Internationale Tagung Vom 20, April bis 24, in Bad Berleberg 231–36.

Furth H (1973) Deafness and Learning: Psychosocial Approach. Ca.: Wadsworth.

Galvin KM, Brommel BJ. (1991) Family Communication, Cohesion and Change, New York, NY: Harper Collins.

Garland DS (1983) Working with Couples for Marriage Enrichment. London: Jossey-Base.

Gilhome-Herbst K (1983) Acquired Deafness in Adults of Employment and Retirement Age, Some Social Implications. PhD Thesis submitted to the London School of Economics and Political Science.

Gilligan C (1982) In a Different Voice. Cambridge, Massachusetts: Harvard University Press.

Gilmore J (1982) Interpersonal Relations and Hearing Loss, HLAS SHHH Self-help for Hearing Impaired People, Beheads, Maryland.

Glennie E (1990) Good Vibrations, Autobiography. London: Hutchinson.

Glickman N (1986) Cultural identity, deafness and mental health. Journal of Rehabilitation of the Deaf 20(2): 1–10.

Goffman E (1963) Stigma. Harmondsworth: Penguin.

Gottlieb BH (1981) Preventive interventions involving social networks and social support. In BH Gottlieb (ed.) Social Networks and Social Support. Beverly Hills: Sage.

Gouldner AW (1960) The norm of reciprocity: a preliminary statement. American Sociological Review 25(2): 161–78.

Greenaway P (2000) Interview with the Chief Scientific Officer of the Department of Health at Skipton House, London, 22 March.

Griffiths P (2000) Letter received from the Course Leader, MSc Counselling in Health Care and Rehabilitation, Brunel University, Department of Health Care Studies, Osterley Campus, Borough Road, Isleworth, Middlesex.

Grimshaw R (1991) Interpretations of children having a parent with complex disabilities, Scottish Concern 19.

Gubrium JF, Holstein JA (1990) What is Family? London: Mayfield Publishing Company.

Handel G (ed.) (1985) The Family as a Mediator of the Culture. The Psychosocial Interior of the Family. New York: Aldine De Gruyter.

Hare-Mustin RT (1978) A feminist approach to family. Therapy Family Process 17: 181–94.

Harris J (1995) The Cultural Meaning of Deafness, Language, Identity and Power. Aldershot: Avebury.

Harvey MA (1989) Psychotherapy with Deaf and Hard of Hearing Persons. London: Lawrence Erbaum Association.

Haskey J (1982) The proportion of marriages ending in divorce. Population Trends 27: 2–11.

Haskey J (1992) Pre-marital Cohabitation and the Probability of Subsequent Divorce: Analyses Using New Data from the General Household Survey, Population Trends. London: HMSO, 10–19.

Hearing News (1992) Croydon Hard of Hearing Project Newsletter. Community Care Office, 1 July.

Hegarty S, Pocklington K, Crowe M (1983) The Making of a Profession: A Study of the Training and Work of the First Hearing Therapists. London: Chameleon Press.

Heller B, Flohr L, Zegan LS (1987) Psychological Interventions with Sensorially Disabled Persons. San Francisco: Grune and Stratton Inc.

Hetu R, Jones L, Getty L (1993) The impact of acquired hearing loss on intimate relationships: implications for rehabilitation. Audiology 32: 363–81.

Higgens P (1980) Outsiders in a Hearing World: A Sociology of Deafness. London: Sage Publications.

Hillery GA (1955) Definitions of community: areas of agreement. Rural Sociology 20: 111–23.

Hill R (1949) Families Under Stress. New York: Harper.

Hoad AD, Oliver MJ, Silver JR (1990) The Experience of Spinal Cord Injury for Other Family Members: A Retrospective Study. London: Thames Polytechnic.

Hockey J, James A (1993) Growing Up and Growing Old, Ageing and Dependency in the Life Course. London: Sage Publications.

Hoffmeister RJ (1985) Families with deaf parents: a functional perspective. In SK Thurman (ed.), Children of Handicapped Parents, Research and Clinical Perspectives. London: Academic Press Inc. 111–30.

Holmes TH, Rahe RH (1967) The Social Readjustment Rating Scale. Journal of Psychosomatic Research 2: 213–18.

Hooglander-Mensink C (1992) Letter received from social worker at the Audiological Institute, Gronigen, Holland.

House JS and Robbins C (1983) Age, psychological stress and health. In M Riley et al. (ed.) Aging in Society. Selected Reviews of Recent Research. Hillsdale, NJ: Lawrence Erlbaum.

Humphrey C, Gilhome-Herbst K, Faurqi S (1981) Some characteristics of the hearing-impaired elderly who do not present themselves for rehabilitation. British Journal of Audiology 15: 25–30.

Huntington J (1982) Migration as part of life experience. Paper given at the New South Wales Institute of Psychiatry. Seminar in Cross Cultural Therapy, October.

Huntington J (1984) Migration as bereavement or expatriate stress and breakdown. Paper Given to Guy's Charter, 2nd Annual Symposium Royal College of Physicians. London, October.

Hunt WM (1944) Progressive deafness. Laryngoscope 54: 229–34.

Hyman HH (1942) The psychology of status. Archives of Psychology 269.

James AL, Wilson K (1986) Couples, Conflict and Change. London: Tavistock Publications.

Jones L (1984) Using drama therapy in research work. Journal for British Association for Drama Therapists 8(1).

Jones L, Kyle J, Wood P (1987) Words apart: losing your hearing as an adult. London: Tavistock Publications.

Joselevich E (1988) Family transitions, cumulative stress, and crises. In C Falicov (ed.), Family Transitions: Continuity and Change Over the Life Cycle. London: The Guilford Press, 273–91.

Jung C (1925) Marriage as a Psychological Relationship in the Development of the Personality Vol. XVIII Collected Works. London: Routledge & Kegan Paul.

Kaplan HS (1979) Disorders of Sexual Desire and Other New Concepts and Techniques in Sex Therapy. London: Bruner/Mazel.

Kazak AE, Marvin RS (1984) Differences, difficulties and adaptation: stress and social networks in families with a handicapped child. In E Earhart, MV Sporakowski (eds), Family Relations, Journal of Applied Family and Child Studies, January, Blacksburg, Virginia: National Council of Family Relations 33: 67–77.

Kent County Social Services, Summary Community Care Plan, Adult and Children's Services, 1993/94–1995/96.

Kiely GM (1984) Social change and marital problems: implications for marriage counselling. British Journal of Guidance and Counselling 12(1): 92–100.

Kisor H (1990) What's That Pig Outdoors. New York: Hill & Wang.

Klein J (1987) Our Need for Others and Its Roots in Infancy. London: Tavistock.

Komarovsky (1962) Blue Collar Marriage. London: Yale University Press.

Kraepelin E (1915) Der Verfolgungswahn der Schwerhoriger, Psychiatric Auflage Leipzig: Barth 8(4).

Krebs DL (1970) Altruism: an examination of concept and a review of the literature, Psychological Bulletin 73: 258–302.

Kubler-Ross E (1970) On Death and Dying. London: The Macmillan Company.

Kyle J (1993) The deafness of psychology. Paper based on a presentation to the London Conference of Psychologists in Deafness, 7 December 1992. In P. Arnold (ed.), Deafness and Development 3(2): February.

Kyle J, Jones L, Wood P (1985) Adjustment to acquired hearing loss: a working model. In H Orlans (ed.), Adjustment to Adult Hearing Loss. London: Taylor & Francis, 119–38.

Lamb ME, Pleck JH, Levine JA (1987) Effects of increased paternal involvement on fathers and mothers. In C Lewis, M O'Brien (eds), Reassessing Fatherhood. London: Sage.

Lamont M, Harris M, Thomas A (1981) Severe Hearing Loss. Department of Applied Social Studies, Polytechnic of North London (unpublished).

Lancet (1994) Epidemic of hearing loss predicted. The Lancet 344 (September): 675.

Lane H (1984) When the Mind Hears, A History of the Deaf. London: Penguin Books.

Larson R, Zuzanek J, Mannell R (1985) Being alone versus being with people: disengagement in daily experience of older adults. Journal of Gerontology 40: 375–81.

Lazarsfeld P, Merton R (1954) Friendship as a social process. In M Berger, T Abee, CH Page (eds), Freedom and Control in Modern Society. Princeton: Van Nostrand.

Leach E (1968) A Runaway World. London: BBC Publications.

Leete R (1979) Changing Patterns of Family Formation and Dissolution in England and Wales 1964-1976. Studies in Medical and Population Subjects No. 39. Office of Population Censuses and Surveys. London: HMSO.

Lenny J (1994) Do disabled people need counselling? In J Swain, V Finkelstein, S French, M Oliver (eds), Disabling Barriers-Enabling Environments. London: Sage Publications, 233–40.

Levene B (1992). Interview with Hearing Therapy's joint course coordinator at the Centre for the Deaf and Speech Therapy, Keeley Street, London on 30 March.

Levene B, Nickolls B, Pryce H (1996) Hearing therapy: a person-centred approach to aural rehabilitation. Journal of the International Federation of Hard of Hearing People 17(2): ISSN 0255-0326, October.

Levine ES (1960) The Psychology of Deafness: Techniques of Appraisal for Rehabilitation. New York: Columbia University Press.

Lewis J, Meredith B (1988) Daughters Who Care. London: Routledge.

Lowenthal MF, Haven B (1968) Interaction and adaptation: intimacy as a critical variable. American Sociological Review 31(1): 22–30.

Lundmark B, Hellstrom M (1989) Offers of Rehabilitation for Hearing Impaired with Employment in Sweden – Case Description. Rehabilitation Schwerhoriger, Ertaubter und Gehorloser Internationale Tagung Vom 20, April bis 24. in Bad Berleburg 240–47.

Lundmark B, Hellstrom M (1992) Letter received from the speech and hearing therapists at the Arbetsmarknadsinstitutet Uppsala, Sweden, May.

Maas HS, Kuypers JA (1974) From Thirty to Seventy. London: Jossey-Bass.

McAllister R, Butler E, Lei T (1973) Patterns of social interaction among families of behaviourally retarded children. Journal of Marriage and Family 35: 93–100.

Mace D (1981) Why marriage enrichment. Marriage Guidance Journal 19(6): 260.

McGhee JC (1985) The effects of siblings on the life satisfaction of the rural elderly. Journal of Marriage and the Family 47: 85–91.

McGoldrick M (1991) Women through the family life cycle. In M McGoldrick, CM Anderson, F Walsh (eds), Women in Families, A Framework for Family Therapy. London: W.W. Norton & Co., 200–26.

McKnight J (1981) Professionalised Service and Disabling Help. In AA Crechin, P Liddiard and J Swain (eds), Handicap in a Social World, Sevenoaks: Hodder & Stoughton in Association with the Open University.

Mansfield P, Collard J (1988) The Beginning of the Rest of Your Life? A Portrait of Newly Wed Marriage. London: Macmillan Press Ltd.

Mansfield P, Collard J. (1991) The couple: a sociological perspective. In W Dryden (ed.), Handbook of Couple Counselling. London: Open University.

Markides A (1983) Denmark as a contemporary European model of aural rehabilitation. In W Watts (ed.), Rehabilitation and Acquired Deafness. Beckenham, Kent: Croom Helm Ltd.

Marris P (1986) Loss and Change. London: Routledge & Kegan Paul.

Marsh P (1987) Social work and fathers. In C Lewis, M O'Brien (eds), Reassessing Fatherhood, New Observations on Fathers and the Modern Family. London: Sage, 183–96.

Martin B (1992) Turning right. Social Work Today 24(2).

Mattinson J (1977) The Reflection Process in Casework Supervision. London: Institute of Marital Studies, The Tavistock Institute of Human Relations.

Mattinson J (1988) Work, Love and Marriage. London: Gerald Duckworth & Co. Ltd.

Mattinson J, Clulow C (1989) Marriage Inside Out: Understanding Problems of Intimacy. London: Penguin.

Mattinson J, Sinclair I (1981) Mate and Stalemate, Institute of Marital Studies. London: Basil Blackwell Ltd.

May C (1992) Individual care? Power and subjectivity in therapeutic relationships. Sociology 26(4): 589–602.

Mensink-Hoolander C. (1992) Letter received from social worker at the Audiological Institute, Groniger, Holland.

Milardo RM (1988) Families and Social Networks. London: Sage Publications.

Montgomery RJV, Gonyea JG, Hooyman NR (1985) Caregivers and the experience of subjective and objective burden. Family Relations 34: 19–25.

Morgan DHJ (1981) Berger and Kellner's construction of marriage. Occasional Paper No. 7, Department of Sociology, University of Manchester, Manchester M13 9PL.

Morgan-Jones RA (1991) Methodology and myth: The impact of hearing impairment on family life. Rehabilitation Schwerhoriger, Ertaubter und Gehorloser 2. Internationale Tagung 21. Marz in Bad Berleburg.

Morgan-Jones RA (1993) Psychosocial components of lip-reading: non cognitive factors. In W Richtberg, K Verch (eds), Help for Hearing Impaired People, Medical and Psychosocial Aspects for Overcoming Hearing Impairments in Various Degrees. Academia: 338–45.

Morgan-Jones RA (1998) Causes of lip-reading stress: some psychosocial factors, Catchword, The Magazine of the Association of Teachers of Lip-reading to Adults. 43 (Autumn): 16–29.

Morris J (1994) Housing, independent living and physically disabled people. In J Swain, V Finklestein, S French, M Oliver (eds), Disabling Barriers-Enabling Environment. London: Sage Publications, 136–44.

Mouser MF, Powers EA, Keith PM, Goudy WJ (1985) Marital status and life satisfaction: a study of older men. In WA Petersen, J Quadagno (eds), Social Bonds in Later Life. London: Sage, 71–90.

Mulrooney J (1973) The Newly-Deafened Adult. Proceedings, National Conference on Program Development for and with Deaf People.

Nemon A (1998) In discussion with at San Francisco State University, San Francisco, Ca. 12 October.

Neugarten B (1972) Personality and the aging process. Gerontologist 12: 9–15.

Nicholls B (1992) The role of the hearing therapist. Network 26 published by the National Association of Deafened People.

Nicholls B (2000) Letter from the Course Co-ordinator, Diploma in Hearing Therapy at the University of Bristol.

Nissel M (1987) Social change and the family cycle. In G Cohen (ed.), Social Change and the Life Course. London: Tavistock Publications Ltd.

Noller P (1984) Nonverbal Communication and Marital Interaction. University of Queensland, Australia: Pergamon Press.

Nussbaum JF, Thompson T, Robinson JD (1989) Communication and Ageing. London: Harper & Row.

O'Brien JE (1985) Network analysis of mid-life transitions: a hypothesis on phases of change in microstructures. In WA Peterson, J Quadagno (eds), Social Bonds in Later Life, Ageing and Interdependence. London: Sage, 143–64.

Oliver M (1983) Social Work with Disabled People. British Association of Social Workers, London: The Macmillan Press Ltd.

Oliver M (1990) The Politics of Disablement. London: Macmillan.

Oliver M, Barnes C (1994) Discrimination, disability and welfare: from needs to rights. In J Swain, V Finkelstein, S French, M Oliver (eds), Disabling Barriers-Enabling Environment. London: Sage Publications 267–77.

Olson DH (1975) Intimacy and Aging Family, Realities of Aging. College of Home Economics, University of Minnesota.

Olson DH (1977) Quest for intimacy. Unpublished paper. University of Minnesota, Minnesota.

Olson DH, Fournier DG, Druckman JM (1986) PREPARE, PREPARE-MC and ENRICH inventories. St Paul, MN:PREPARE/ENRICH, Inc.

Olson DH, Lavee Y, McCubbin HI (1988) Types of families and family responses to stress across the family life cycle. In DM Klein, J Aldous (eds), Social Stress and Family Development. London: The Guilford Press, 16–43.

Olson DH, McCubbin HC, Barnes H, Larsen A, Muxen M, Wilson M (1983) Families, What Makes Them Work. Beverly Hills, CA: Sage.

Olson D, Sprenkle D, Russell C (1979) Circumplex model of marital and family systems: cohesion and adaptability dimension, family types and clinical application. Family Process 18: 3–28.

Olson DH, Wilson WA (1982) Family Satisfaction Scale. In DH Olson, HI McCubbin, HL Barnes, AS Larsen, MJ Muxen, Wilson (eds), Family Inventories. St Paul: Family Social Science, University of Minnesota.

One Plus One (1998)The Marriage and Partnership Research Charity, London: One Plus One Information Pack, Spring.

Orlans H (1985) Adjustment to Adult Hearing Loss, London: Taylor & Francis.

Oyer HJ, Oyer EJ (1985) Adult hearing loss and the family. In H Orlans (ed.), Adjustment to Adult Hearing Loss. San Diego: College Hill Press, 139–54.

Oyer and Paolucci B (1970) Homemakers' hearing loss and family integration. Journal of Home Economics 62: 257–62.

Padden C (1989) Interview with Professor of Communication at the University of California, San Diego on 28 August.

Padden C, Humphries T (1988) Deaf in America, Voices from a Culture. London: Harvard University Press.

Park RE (1950) Race and Culture. Glencoe, Il: The Free Press, vi–vii.

Parker G (1993) With This Body, Caring and Disability in Marriage. Buckingham: Open University Press.

Parkes CM (1987) Bereavement, Studies of Grief in Adult Life. Harmondsworth: Penguin Books.

Parkes CM, Weiss RS (1983) Recovery from Bereavement. New York: Basic Books.

Parrott D (1992) A Service to the 17 per cent: A Study of Ideology and Deafness Work in Social Service Departments. Thesis submitted in fulfilment of the requirements for the degree of Doctor of Philosophy in the School of Social Studies, University of Essex.

Parsons T, Bales R (1955) Family Socialisation and Interaction Process. Glencoe Illinois: Free Press.

Paxman J (1998) The English. London: Penguin Books.

Perlman D (1988) Loneliness: a life-span family perspective. In RM Milardo (ed.), Families and Social Networks. London: Sage Publications.

Phillipson C (1987) The transition to retirement. In G Cohen (ed.), Social Change and the Life Course. London: Tavistock Publications.

Pincus L (1974) Death and the Family, The Importance of Mourning. London: Faber & Faber.

Pittman FS (1988) Family crises: expectable and unexpectable. In CJ Falicov (ed.), Family Transitions, Continuity and Change over the Life Cycle. London: The Guilford Press, 255–71.

Preston P (1994) Mother Father Deaf, Living Between Sound and Silence. London: Harvard University Press.

Quine L, Pahl J (1985) Families with Mentally Handicapped Children: A Study of Stress and Service Response. Health Service Research Unit, University of Kent at Canterbury.

Rabbit P (1986) Cognitive effect of mild deafness. Soundbarrier. London: RNID, June.

Rapoport R, Rapoport RN (1971) Dual-Career Families. Harmondsworth: Penguin.

Rapoport R, Rapoport RN (1975) Leisure and the Family Life Cycle. London: Routledge & Kegan Paul.

Rapoport R, Rapoport RN (eds) (1978) Working Couples. London: Routledge & Kegan Paul.

Rapoport R, Rapoport RN, Strelitz Z (1977) Fathers, Mothers, and Others. London: Routledge & Kegan Paul.

Rawson A (1973) The Rawson Report. London.

Ree J (1999) I See a Voice. London: Harper & Collins.

Reis H, Wheeler L, Spiegel N, Kernis M, Nezlek J, Perri M (1982) Physical attractiveness in social interaction II: why does appearance affect social experience? Journal of Personality and Social Psychology 43: 979–96.

Reiss D (1981) The Family's Construction of Reality. London: Harvard University Press.

Ridgeway S (1991) Deaf Mental Health Professionals - Necessary or Token. Paper delivered at the Mental Health and Deafness Conference, St George's Hospital, Tooting, 15 November.

Roberto KA, Scott IP (1986) Equity consideration in the friendships of older adults, Journal of Gerontology 41: 241–7.

Romano M (1984) The impact of disability on family and society. In JV Basmajian (ed.), Foundations of Medical Rehabilitation. Baltimore: Williams and Wilkens.

Rosen S, Bergman M, Plester D, El-Mofty A, Satti M (1982) Presbyacusis Study of a Relatively Noise Free Population in the Sudan. Annuals of Otology, Rhinology and Laryngology 71:727–43.

Rosnow I (1967) Social Integration of the Aged. New York: Free Press.

Rosow I (1957) Issues in the concept of need-complementarity, Sociometry 20 (September): 216–33.

Royal National Institute of the Deaf (1996) Statistics Relating to Deafness.

Royal National Institute for the Deaf Research Group (1990) Statistics Relating to Deafness. October.

Rubel EW (1994) Hair Cell Regeneration: We've Come a Long Way in a Few Short Years. The John Hopkins University Symposium: Focus on Research, New Discoveries, New Solutions. The Ninth International Meeting of SHHH, Baltimore, Maryland.

Sacks O (1990) Seeing Voices. London: Picado.

Safilios-Rothschild C (1970) The Sociology and Social Psychology of Disability and Rehabilitation. Washington D.C.: University Press of America.

Sainsbury S (1970) Registered as Disabled. Occasional Papers on Social Administration No. 35. London: Bell and Sons.

Sainsbury S (1986) Deaf Worlds. London: Hutchinson and Co.

Sainsbury S (1993) In discussion with on 17 March at the London School of Economics.

Sarason IG (1980) Test Anxiety, Theory, Research and Application. Hillside N.J.: Lawrence Erlbaum Associates.

Satir V (1972) Peoplemaking. Norwich: Fletcher and Son.

Scanzoni J, Plonko K, Teachman J, Thompson L (1989) The Sexual Bond, Rethinking Families and Close Relationships. London: Sage.

Scanzoni L, Scanzoni J (1981) Men, Women, and Change. New York: McGraw Hill.

Schachter J (1959) The Psychology of Affiliation. Stanford, CA: Stanford University Press.

Schaefer MT, Olson D (1981) Assessing intimacy: The PAIR Inventory. Journal of Marital and Family Therapy 7: 47–60.

Schiff-Meyers NB (1982) Sign and oral language development of preschool children of deaf parents in comparison with their mother's communication system, American Annals of the Deaf 127: 322–30.

Schilling F, Gilchrist LD, Schinke SP (1984) Coping and social support in families of developmentally disabled children. Family Relations, Journal of Applied Family Studies. Published by the National Council on Family Relations 33(1):47–54.

Schlesinger H (1985) The psychology of hearing loss. In H Orlans (ed.), Adjustment to Adult Hearing Loss. London: Taylor & Francis, 99–118.

Schlesinger H (1986) Reliance on Self and Others: Autonomy and the Lessening of Dependency of Young Deaf Adults. Regional Conference on Postsecondary Education for Hearing Impaired Persons, Postsecondary Consortium, The University of Tennessee.

Schloch R (1988) Relations and Communication Between Well Hearing and Hearing Impaired. Third International Congress of the Hard of Hearing 3–8 July, Montreux, Switzerland: Buchdruckerei Richterswil AG, CH-8805 Richterswil 290–2.

Scott RA (1969) The Making of Blind Men: A Study of Adult Socialisation. New York: Russell Sage.

Segal J, Simkins J (1993) My Mum Needs Me, Helping Children with Ill or Disabled Parents. London: Penguin Books.

Segal L (ed.) (1983) What is to Be Done about the Family. Harmondsworth: Penguin.

SHHH (1983) Self Help in Action: Special Report. Bethesda, Maryland: SHHH Publications.

SHHH (1989) Living Alone with a Hearing Loss. SHHH Information Series # 201, Bethesda, Maryland: SHHH Publications.

SHHH (1999) Young Children in Families with a Parent with Hearing Loss. Bethesda, Maryland: SHHH Publications 16–18.

Sleeboom-van Raaij CJ (1993) Sudden deafness and psychiatric assistance. In W Richtberg, Klaus Verch (eds), Help for Hearing Impaired People, Medical and Psychosocial Aspects for Overcoming Hearing Impairments in its Various Degrees. Sankt Augustin: Academia Verlag, 384–6.

Sloss Luey H (1980) Between worlds: the problems of deafened adults. Social Work in Health Care 5: 253–65.

Sloss Luey H (1992) Letter from research associate, Adult Onset Hearing Loss Project, University of California San Francisco, Ca.

Sloss Luey H (2000) Letter from the Director of the San Francisco Hearing Society, San Francisco, Ca.

SSA Magazine (1993) Men in families: new roles, new challenges. The School of Social Service Administration, The University of Chicago 5 (1) (Fall): 3–5.

Stein G (1935) The Gradual Making of The Making of Americans. Lectures in America. New York: Random House.

Sternberg RJ (1986) A triangular theory of love. Psychological Review 93(2): 119–35.

Stevens E (1966) Churchill as patient: his relaxed attitude towards his deafness. Letter in the Daily Telegraph, 24 June.

Strain LA, Chappel NL (1982) Confidants: do they make a difference in the quality of life. Researching on Aging 4: 479–502.

Sullivan, HS (1953) The Interpersonal Theory of Psychiatry. New York: Norton.

Sussman A (1986) Psychotherapy and Deafness. Course, Fremont School for the Deaf, Fremont. Ca.

Suttles G (1970) Friendship as a Social Institution. In G McCall (ed.) Social Relationships. Chicago: Aldine.

Sutton-Smith B and Rosenberg BG (1970) The Siblings. New York: Holt Rinehart & Winston.

Swain J, Finkelstein V, French S, Oliver M (ed) (1994) Disabling Barriers-Enabling Environments. London: Sage Publications in Association with the Open University.

Tannen D (1986) 'That's Not What I Meant': How Conversation Style Makes or Breaks Relationships. New York: Ballantine Books.

Tannen D (1989) Talking Voices, Repetition, Dialogue, and Imagery in Conversational Discourse. Cambridge: Cambridge University Press.

Tannen D (1991) You Just Don't Understand. New York: Ballantine Books.

Thomas AJ (1984) Acquired Hearing Loss: Psychological and Psychosocial Implications. London: Academic Press.

Thomas AJ, Herbst KG (1980) Social and psychological implications of acquired deafness in adults of employment age. British Journal of Audiology 14: 76–85.

Thornes B, Collard J (1979) Who Divorces? London: Routledge & Kegan Paul.

Thunem J (1966) The invalid mind. In P Hunt (ed.), Stigma. London: Geoffrey Chapman.

Thurman SK (ed.) (1985) Children of Handicapped Parents. Research and Clinical Perspectives. London: Academic Press Inc.

Townsend P (1963) The Family Life of Old People. London: Pelican.

Townsend P (1979) Poverty in the United Kingdom. Harmondsworth: Penguin.

Troll LE (1971) The family of later life: a decade review. Journal of Marriage and the Family 33: 263–90.

Unger DG, Powell DR (1980) Supporting families under stress: the role of social networks. Family Relations 29: 566–74.

Ungerson C (1987) Policy is Personal: Sex, Gender, and Informal Care. London: Tavistock.

van Dongen-Garrad J (1983) Invisible Barriers: Pastoral Care with the Physically Disabled. London: SPCK.

Vernon M, Griffin D, Yoken C (1982) Hearing Loss: Problems in Family Practice,# HLAS7. SHHH Information Leaflets, Bethesda, Maryland.

Vernon M, Makowsky B (1969) Deafness and minority group dynamics. The Deaf American July/August, 3–6.

von der Leith L (1972) Experimental social deafness. Scandinavian Audiology 1: 1–87.

von der Leith L (1993) Auswertung Der Tagung und Schlusswort. 3 Internationale Tagung Rehabilitation Schwerhoriger, Ertaubter und Gehorloser, April 22–6, Bad Berlberg, Germany.

Voysey M (1975) A Constant Burden, the Reconstruction of Family Life. London: Routledge & Kegan Paul.

Walsh F (1998) Strengthening Family Resilience. London: Guilford Press.

Walsh F, McGoldrick M. (1988) Loss and the family life cycle. In CJ Falicov (ed.), Family Transitions. London: The Guilford Press, 311–36.

Walsh F, McGoldrick M. (1991) Living Beyond Loss, Death in the Family. London: W.W. Norton & Co.

Warnes A (1993) Being old, old people, and the burdens of burden Ageing and Society 13(3): 297–338.

Wax T (1989) Assessment dilemmas of late-onset hearing loss. In H Sloss Luey, H Elliott, L Glass (eds), Mental Health Assessment of Deaf Clients. Proceedings of a conference: 12 and 13 February, San Francisco, Ca.

Webb HW (1989) The pastor's opportunities XXVI: Ministry to the Hearing Impaired. The Expository Times 100(9): 328–32.

Weingarten K (1978) Interdependence. In R Rapoport, RN Rapoport (eds), Working Couples. London: Routledge & Kegan Paul, 147–8.

Wheeler D, Avis JM, Miller LA, Chaney R (1991) Rethinking family therapy training and supervision: a feminist model. In McGoldrick M, Anderson M, Walsh F (eds), Women in Families. London: WW Norton & Co., 135–65.

Willi J (1982) Couples in Collusion: The Unconscious Dimension in Partner Relationships. Claremont California: Hunter House.

Willmott P (1986) Social Networks Informal Care and Public Policy. London: Policy Studies Institute.

Wolff S (1991) Children under stress in a disabled family: an overview. In Scottish Concern, Journal of the National Children's Bureau Scottish Group 19: 24–30.

Wood P (1993) Searching for a model: the dilemma of social rehabilitation in acquired hearing loss. In W Richtberg and K Verch (eds) Help for Hearing Impaired People. Sankt Augustin: Academia Verlag, 384–7.

Wood PL, Kyle J, Jones L (1983) Hearing Aid Use and Level of Support for People Who Become Deaf. Bristol: School of Education Research Unit, University of Bristol.

Woods JC (1986) Lip-reading, A Guide for Beginners. London: RNID.

Woolley M (1994) Acquired hearing loss: acquired oppression. In J Swain, V Finkelstein, S French, M Oliver, Disabling Barriers – Enabling Environments. London: Sage Publications.

Wright D (1990) Deafness, A Personal Account. London: Faber & Faber.

Wynne LC (1988) An epigenetic model of family processes. In CJ Falicov (ed.) Family Transitions: Continuity and Change over the Life Cycle. London: The Guilford Press, 81–106.

Young M, Willmott P (1972) The Symmetrical Family, A Study of Work and Leisure in the London Region. Harmondsworth: Penguin.

Index

699205